**Yoga for chronic pain in veterans:
A mixed methods study**

Melvin Turner Donaldson

© Melvin Turner Donaldson 2018

B: TABLE OF CONTENTS

A: Abstract	ii
B: Table of Contents	v
C: List of Tables	vii
D: List of Figures	viii
E: Population burden of chronic pain	1
E.1. Standard of care treatments are inadequate for most	2
E.2. Resilience in chronic pain	3
F: Yoga for chronic pain	6
F.1. What is yoga?	6
F.2. Potential mechanisms for the effect of yoga in chronic pain	8
G: Conceptual model of study	11
G.1. Model of effect of yoga on pain interference	12
G.2. Model of relationship of mode and maintenance of yoga practice	14
G.3. Operationalizing resilience and vulnerability coping factors	19
H: Research Questions and Significance	24
I: Study Design	29
I.1. Overview of study	29
I.2. Description of RINGS-CAM study	30
I.3. Measures	34
Manuscript 1: Cross-sectional association of yoga practice and interfering pain	38
J.1. Introduction	38
J.2. Methods	40
J.3. Results	47
J.4. Discussion	49
J.5. Tables and Figures	52
Manuscript 2: How pain shapes the experience of yoga among veterans: A mixed methods study	57
K.1. Introduction	57
K.2. Methods	58
K.3. Results	66

K.4.	Discussion	76
K.5.	Tables and Figures	80

MANUSCRIPT 3: PATTERNS OF USE OF NON-PHARMACOLOGICAL HEALTH PRACTICES . 90

L.1.	Introduction	90
L.2.	Methods	93
L.3.	Results	101
L.4.	Discussion	105
L.5.	Tables and Figures	112

M: DISCUSSION AND SUMMARY ... 123

M.1.	Summary of results	123
M.2.	Conceptual models	126
M.3.	Discussion	128

N: BIBLIOGRAPHY ... 132

C: LIST OF TABLES

Table G-1: Proposed pain resilience and vulnerability factors. 19

Table J-1: Characteristics of complete case analysis sample 52

Table J-2: Bivaraite associations of characteristics and pain interference 53

Table J-3: Bivariate associations of characteristics and yoga practice 54

Table J-4: Balance of covariates after propensity score matching 55

Table K-1: Semi-structured interview guide 81

Table K-2: Characteristics of survey participants 82

Table K-3: Characteristics of yoga practitioners with and without chronic pain .. 83

Table K-4: Essential Properties of Yoga Questionnaire Part 1 84

Table K-5: Essential Properties of Yoga Questionnaire Part 2. 85

Table K-6: Emergent themes (6) from the qualitative analysis 86

Table K-7: Characteristics of interview participants 87

Table L-1: Self-reported past-year use of Health Practices 112

Table L-2: Comparison of model fit statistics 114

Table L-3: Characteristics of respondents to the mailed survey 115

Table L-4: Probability of use of Health Practices Inventory approaches 116

Table L-5: Characteristics of survey respondents and non-respondents 121

Table L-6: Prevalence differences of class membership due to covariates 122

D: LIST OF FIGURES

Figure G-1: Model of the impact of yoga practice on chronic pain 12

Figure G-2: Model of relationship between mode and maintentnace of yoga 18

Figure I-1: Items of the PHQ-8 34

Figure I-2: PCL-5 20 items 35

Figure I-3: DAST-10 items 36

Figure I-4: Alcohol Use Disorders Identification Test (AUDIT) items 37

Figure J-1: 7 items of the Graded Chronic Pain Scale (GCPS) and scoring 56

Figure K-1: Mixed methods design schematic of this study 80

Figure K-2: Full Text of the Essential Properties of Yoga Questionnaire 88

Figure L-1: Table of effect of covariates on prevalence of latent classes 118

Figure L-2: Full text of the Health Practices Inventory 119

Figure M-1: Updated, integrated conceptual model 131

viii

E: POPULATION BURDEN OF CHRONIC PAIN

Chronic pain is a significant public health problem in the US. It is highly prevalent: over 100 million Americans are estimated to experience chronic pain at any given time.[1] It is costly. Conservative estimates place measurable loss in productivity and direct costs due to chronic pain at over $500 billion annually.[1] It can be debilitating. For the past 25 years, back and neck pain have been the second leading cause of disease burden in wealthy nations.[2] Low back pain is the leading cause of disability globally.[3,4] Yet pain is still poorly managed. Trends over the past decade in the United States indicate that chronic pain is increasingly being managed with guideline-discordant rather than evidence-based approaches.[5] Additionally, US soldiers and veterans experience chronic pain at a higher prevalence and with worse outcomes than in the general US population.[6–11]

Pain is an evolutionarily ancient physiological phenomenon that changes an organism's behavior in the presence of potential tissue damage. Pain can be useful for discovering otherwise hidden injury. The first step in the management of pain is the identification (or ruling out) of a specific anatomical cause.[12,13] Cancer, infection, fractures and anatomical abnormalities are a few broad categories of causes of bone and joint pain that have specific medical management that would be considered.

Chronic pain is a general term used when a patient experiences continuous or recurrent pain for an extended time. Definitions have been variable in both clinical medicine and research[14,15] but consensus is moving towards a definition for chronic pain of pain that occurs most days for at least six months.[16] The most common[14] chronic pain complaints in US adults are low back pain, headache, and neck pain. Only rarely is chronic pain at one of these most common sites associated with an identifiable abnormality.[13] In some patients, the constellation of pain sites and associated symptoms is better described by a particular chronic pain condition[15] such as fibromyalgia or temporomandibular joint dysfunction; however, multiple co-morbid pain conditions is common. Moreover, it is unclear that distinct chronic pain conditions represent distinct disease processes.

E.1.   Standard of care treatments are inadequate for most

Many pharmacological agents are available for pain, and a number are specifically recommended (e.g. in low back pain) yet their efficacy and safety profiles vary widely.[12] Any given drug therapy is at best moderately effective for a minority of chronic pain patients.[17–21] Recommended drug classes include acetaminophen (i.e. Tylenol), non-steroidal anti-inflammatories (NSAIDs: e.g., ibuprofen, naproxen, ketorolac) and tricyclic antidepressants (TCAs: e.g. amitriptyline, nortriptyline). Little is known about predicting the most effective drug for any given patient and none of the effective drugs are considered definitive treatment for the pain. The established harms of opioid therapy[22–24] together with evidence of no higher effectiveness than non-opioid therapies[25] has resulted in changing prescribing guidelines.[14] This creates an important need for other options.[26–28]

E.2. Resilience in chronic pain

Resilience as a construct on its own is generally used to describe people who "do well" despite perturbations.[29] Sturgeon & Zautra propose using a specific definition in the context of pain: resilient individuals experience low levels of pain interference in the presence of high levels of pain severity.[30] In this sense, resilience factors moderate the relationship between a stressor (pain) and return to normal (homeostasis). This does not necessarily mean that resilience requires significant stressors (a high allostatic load) but measuring resilience might necessitate that. One paradigm in resilience research posits that resilience is a natural trait of humans and that loss of resilience is pathological.[29] Much of the resilience literature is focused on psychological development and maintaining positive health outcomes as adults in the face of childhood trauma.[31]

The way an individual copes with pain modifies his or her likelihood of experiencing resilient outcomes for pain. Coping strategies are the "specific efforts that people employ to master, tolerate, reduce, or minimize stressful events."[32] This includes cognitive processes, affect/distress and behaviors,[30] as well as one's relationships with others.[33] Here, the particular coping strategies people employ are described as either resilience or vulnerability factors. Resilience factors promote resilient outcomes and vulnerability factors hinder resilient outcomes. Some resilience and vulnerability factors are technical skills that may be taught, learned and mastered. People inherently use a variety of both resilience and vulnerability mechanisms.

Differential coping strategies have been described in a variety of ways in the literature but these distinctions have not been especially useful in understanding outcomes in pain.[32] One distinction is to separate coping strategies as adaptive versus maladaptive. This dichotomy is defined in a rather recursive way: identification of adaptive patterns of coping depends on their association with particular desirable health behaviors and outcomes, as is the case for maladaptive patterns and undesirable behaviors and outcomes.[34] This definition is problematic because the dichotomy is context-dependent: an adaptive coping strategy in one situation may be maladaptive in another. For example, avoidance coping strategies may be adaptive for youth under chronic stress,[35] but avoidant coping strategies have been shown to lead to worse outcomes in the context of chronic pain.[36] Another distinction is to separate behavioral or problem-focused coping strategies from cognitive or emotion-focused strategies, which separates a person's attempts to control the stressor itself (primary control: problem-focused) from a person's attempts to control how she or he feels about or conceptualizes the stressor (secondary control: emotion-focused).[37] This distinction is helpful when a stressor may be identified as controllable or not, but is less helpful in the context of non-specific chronic low back pain as the controllable and uncontrollable aspects of the experience may be inseparable.

In the transactional model of stress appraisal and coping,[38] the strategies individuals use to cope with stressors influences their ultimate outcomes. Their appraisal of the stressor, or how it is perceived, is as important or more important than any objective measure of the impact of the stressor. In the context of pain, this would mean that the way a person with chronic pain perceives the impact of pain in their life could be more important than an objective measure of the severity or intensity of that pain in terms of their ultimate outcomes for pain.

Many people experience stable pain for very long periods of time (years to decades) and in response the nervous system adapts[39]; in the resilience literature, attention is shifted from homeostasis (maintenance) towards a multi-component view of outcomes. Resilient pain outcomes are of three classes: recovery from the episode and returning to equilibrium; sustainability: continuing worthwhile life pursuits in the face of pain stressors; and growth, which is a continual process of learning the extent of one's capabilities.[40] Theorized markers of resilient outcomes include low levels of depression and anxiety following a personal loss (recovery), maintaining elevated positive emotion and hope in the presence of a stressor (sustainability) and lower levels of depression and more elevated positive emotion than before the stressor (growth). In this sense, the outcome classes are latent constructs that are not directly measurable,[40] although several scales have been developed that quantify different aspects of growth, in the context of "posttraumatic growth."[40(fig15.1)]

F: YOGA FOR CHRONIC PAIN

Yoga is an increasingly common technique used in the management of chronic back pain.[41] Contemporary yoga practices are multi-modal, integrating the practice of distinct techniques including relaxation, meditation, biofeedback, stretching and exercise.[42] Even though the mechanisms of the effect of yoga on pain are not understood, yoga is a recommended adjunctive therapy to standard of care practices in numerous conditions including chronic low back pain,[13] depression,[43] and hypertension[44] based on demonstrated effectiveness. An estimated 10% of American adults practice yoga,[45] a number which has been steadily increasing over the past decade.[46,47] Yoga appears to be more common among people with chronic pain than among those without.[48,49]

F.1. What is yoga?

Contemporary yoga practice is a comprehensive system of lifestyle guidance that is rooted in the ancient Vedic traditions of India.[50] Physical yoga practice [*asana* in the Sanskrit writings of Patanjali] is one of the major components of the system. Practitioners move their bodies into and out of specific postures and poses with intention and attention to how they feel in the postures as well as how they feel about the process. There are many branches and schools of yoga today, highlighting the different facets of the Vedic teachings with modern iterations.[51–53] Each of these practices uses a combination of *asana* along with mindfulness [*dharana*] or meditation [*dhyana*], breath work [*pranayama*]. Several major modern branches which are relevant to healthcare today include Iyengar, vinyasa, kundalini, viniyoga and Bikram. There is a wide variety in practitioner experiences within these styles. Some of these styles are more athletic than others, some incorporate long periods of stillness and meditation, some have strict standards for instructor development and training. It is unclear what aspects of these practices would make any of them more beneficial for chronic pain than others. Additionally, more athletic styles could seem inaccessible to large groups of people and practices that are particularly dogmatic or have a strong vernacular tradition may seem inaccessible to an equally sizeable group. Potentially, the most important aspect is developing self-discipline [*tapas*] to maintain a regular practice, regardless of the type of yoga practiced. At present, there is no evidence of particular styles of yoga being more beneficial than others.[54]

Yoga intervention research suffers from a problem of effect identification. It is not always clear what authors consider "yoga" versus "not yoga" in their publications[55,56] yet the beneficial effects may be extrapolated to "yoga." Since the definition of yoga varies, the effects of yoga do not have a consistent meaning. Possibly the effects of yoga are mediated by components that make it similar to other effective interventions, not the components that distinguish yoga. Current scholarly work on the effective components of yoga is based on expert opinion.[57,58]

Hypothesized mechanisms of yoga in pain conditions involve the physiologic stress response and autonomic nervous system, brain changes, and physical activity and stretching.[42,59,60] Research in yoga has demonstrated effects on the autonomic nervous system, including relaxation of the sympathetic nervous system (SNS) and hypothalamic-pituitary-adrenal axis (HPAA), major mediators of the neuroendocrine stress response.[61] Yoga practice has been shown to broadly decrease physiologic arousal, decreasing activity of the SNS and HPAA, which is implicated in the calming, relaxing effect of yoga.[62] Dysregulation of the autonomic nervous system appears to play a key role in chronic pain.[63] Arousal of the autonomic nervous system is related to how a person perceives a painful stimulus.[63] In animal models, physical activity has been shown to interrupt the development of persistent pain through its effect on autonomic dysregulation.[63]

F.2. Potential mechanisms for the effect of yoga in chronic pain

VA hospitals around the country offer mind-body practices as a component of comprehensive pain management efforts, including groups in many styles of yoga and mindfulness.[64] "Mind-body" refers to individual or group practices that recognize an integral connection of mind and body and use intentional movement or intentional stillness as a means to facilitate introspection and focus on the present. There is strong evidence that some mind-body practices are modestly or moderately effective in the management of chronic pain.[65] Specifically, several styles of yoga have been shown to help a variety of specific pain conditions.

Encouraging awareness of the dynamic connection of the physical body and subject mind differentiates yoga from other health interventions such as physical exercise at a gym or cognitive behavioral therapy, which focus on isolated components of the mind-body connection; however, physical exercise[66,67] and cognitive behavioral therapy[68] are both also effective in chronic pain management. It is unclear if yoga is effective in the treatment of chronic pain for the same or different reasons as physical exercise or cognitive behavioral therapy.

One of the first US randomized controlled trials to test the effect of a yoga intervention in the treatment of chronic pain showed a better improvement in the yoga arm than a stretching active control arm[69]; the authors suggested that the benefits of yoga may be in part due to mental focus, but that this effect would be difficult to parse out without better understanding of the mechanisms. A later study[70] by the same authors reported no significant difference between yoga and stretching on back pain-related dysfunction and concluded that the benefits of yoga are likely due to stretching rather than any psychological changes. The latter[70] of the two studies was guided by a conceptual framework[71(fig1)] that posited several possible mechanisms for the effect of yoga. In order to examine the importance of the various potential mechanisms proposed, the authors performed a mediation analysis of the trial results.[72] They found that "total hours of back exercise" alone was only responsible for about 10–15% of the total effect of the yoga intervention arm or the stretching control arm.

Unfortunately, this type of theory-driven approach is notably rare in the field and there is no standard way of comparing yoga interventions to other effective interventions along shared components. Until recently, there has been no standard way of even describing the components of yoga interventions.[73] The field would benefit from a standardized framework that would allow investigators to test the effects of components of yoga practice on measurable health outcomes. Examining which components of yoga are responsible for (and necessary for) its effect in pain could lead to improved delivery of yoga or the development of more effective integrated interventions. Additionally, we have an incomplete understanding of what yoga practitioners actually do as a part of their yoga practice outside of interventions. The standardized framework could facilitate pragmatic population studies of how components of yoga benefit real-world practitioners.

G: **CONCEPTUAL MODEL OF STUDY**

I propose that the effect of yoga practice on pain resilience is through its effect on key vulnerability and resilience factors (cognitive appraisal, psychological distress, and change in pain-related behavior), in addition to any independent effect on underlying anatomic abnormalities. To guide this study, I developed a preliminary conceptual model of the hypothesized impact of yoga practice on chronic pain (Figure G-1, p. 12). This conceptual model is based on the theory that a regular yoga practice may foster resilience in individuals with chronic low back pain by helping them develop cognitive and psychological tools to deal with the stress of pain. In the proposed conceptual model, chronic pain resilience is defined as the absence of chronic pain-related functional impairment in the presence of chronic pain.[30,74,75] Subjective pain intensity is a weak predictor of pain-related functional impairment.[76] On the other hand, subjective pain intensity may predict adoption of yoga practice.[48] Compared to the general US population, yoga practitioners have more baseline chronic pain and more medical complaints[77,78]; however, evidence also suggests that yoga practice is associated with reduced risk of interfering chronic pain.[79(p34)] If yoga practitioners have more pain but less interference from pain than non-yoga practitioners, yoga may be associated with pain resilience.

G.1. Model of effect of yoga on pain interference

Figure G-1: Conceptual model of the impact of yoga practice on chronic pain

[Figure G-1: Diagram showing Chronic Pain and Yoga practice leading through Vulnerability & resilience factors (Cognitive appraisal & Personality, Psychological Distress, Pain-related Behaviors) to Disability/Interference]

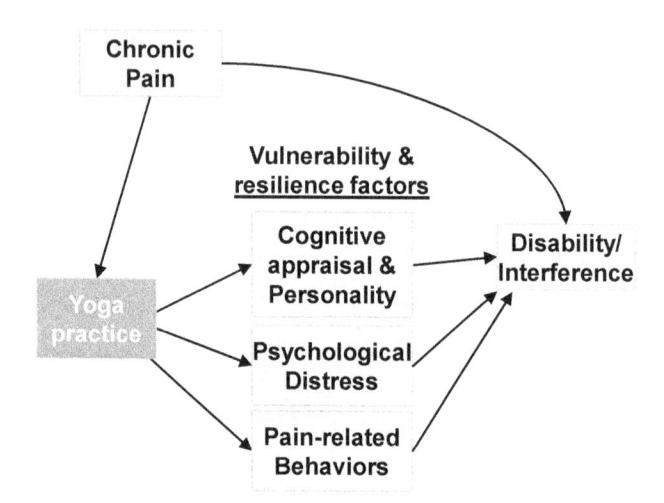

Figure G-1 presents potential vulnerability and resilience pathways through which regular yoga practice may lead to pain resilience among individuals experiencing chronic pain. My conceptual model hypothesizes that through a regular yoga practice, the person experiencing pain learns to think differently about pain (i.e., change in cognitive appraisal) and respond differently to pain (i.e., reduced psychological distress and reduced maladaptive pain-related behavior). Cognitive appraisal, psychological distress, pain-related behaviors, and personality have been shown to be associated with interfering chronic pain.[80] Cognitive appraisal of pain, or how individuals perceive and think about their pain,[81(p111)] includes pain acceptance,[82] catastrophizing,[83] and self-management beliefs.[84] Pain acceptance has been shown to be negatively correlated with pain interference,[85] whereas catastrophizing has been positively correlated with interference.[86] Psychological distress includes depressive[87] and traumatic symptoms[88] that are positively associated with disabling back pain.[89] Finally, externalizing pain-related behaviors including illicit substance use[90] and alcohol use[91] have been shown to be associated with poor functional status.[92] The relative importance of the resilience and vulnerability factors listed above remains elusive. Sociodemographic factors, including age, sex and gender, educational attainment, and combat experience potentially confound the relationship between yoga practice and interfering pain so will be considered in my analyses.

      There is some specific evidence for how yoga practitioners are different from those who don't regularly practice yoga in their perception of pain. Villemure et al. studied pain tolerance in a group of yoga practitioners and a group of yoga-naïve individuals.[93] Yoga practitioners had an increased tolerance to a cold pressor test (time subject tolerates hand in ice water bath) and employed different cognitions (mental strategies) during the experience. The yoga practitioners were more likely to "relax," "accept," "observe" the pain stress or to "breathe" during the cold pressor test. In the parlance of my model, yoga practitioners use resilience coping mechanisms when faced with a noxious stimulus when non-yoga practitioners used vulnerability mechanisms faced with the same stimulus. Additionally, immediately following yoga classes, yoga practitioners were shown to have significantly improved mood, including reporting feeling more "happy," "relaxed," "optimistic," "confident" and "content" compared to before the practice[94]. Yoga practitioners develop their resilience resources through their practice. Finally, in a trial of people with chronic low back pain, after 12 weeks of yoga fewer participants in the intervention group used opiates or other analgesics in response to pain.[95]

Does yoga instill these resilience resources in yoga practitioners or do they come to yoga already possessing these resources? Evidence is limited. Some vulnerability resources predispose people with chronic pain to have negative attitudes towards yoga. People who score high on catastrophizing and kinesiophobia scales are more likely to have negative attitudes toward yoga.[96] Interestingly, yoga may actually benefit people with these vulnerability resources more than others because they would potentially experience the greatest changes in balance of resilience resources in favor of their vulnerability resources. Catastrophizing was associated with low mindfulness in a survey of 104 Australians with chronic pain.[97] An 8-week yoga intervention among women with fibromyalgia showed a significant improvement in pain catastrophizing in the treatment arm.[98] Yoga is recommended as an effective adjunctive treatment for depression, PTSD and occupational stress.[99] Fully understanding the direction of effect between yoga and the resilience and vulnerability resources will require well-designed longitudinal studies.

G.2. Model of relationship of mode of yoga practice with maintenance of practice

Yoga practitioners may generally be practicing independently by themselves, with an instructor, or both. To date, no evidence has emerged to explain the relative importance of these modes of practice in health outcomes or other perceived benefits. Though there may be facilitators and barriers of yoga practice broadly speaking, there may also be a unique subset of facilitators and barriers for the independent and instructor-led modes of practice. Figure G-2 (p. 18) shows the model of the relationship between facilitators and barriers of yoga practice and maintenance of yoga practice. This model is informed by 2 other conceptual models that were presented in 2 qualitative studies of barriers and facilitators to yoga practice.

The first study[100] was conducted with the participants of a randomized trial[101] of yoga for back pain among predominantly low-income, diverse adults in Boston, MA. In their model, potential yoga practitioners (intervention participants) experience facilitators and barriers to attending yoga class. Facilitators of attending class include trusting teachers, the camaraderie with classmates and external support from family. Barriers to attending class include logistics, fear of injuring oneself in class and a lack of motivation. When the balance of facilitators and barriers is in favor to attending class, practitioners go to class. When practitioners attend class, they may perceive benefits from their practice, including enhanced mood, reductions in pain, increased self-confidence, and spiritual effects. These perceived benefits in turn act as an additional facilitator of attending class and act to decrease a lack of motivation barrier to attending class. The model creates yoga practice as a feed-forward loop that encourages further practice.

The second study[102] was conducted to inform methods to enhance participation in an upcoming randomized trial. In the model, certain characteristics of potential yoga practitioners (intervention participants), including their gender, race and ethnicity, religion, age, and socioeconomic status lead to an increased use of "health promoting behaviors," which specifically are attending yoga class and practicing at home. The relationship between participant characteristics and yoga practice is moderated by (weakened or strengthened by) numerous factors, presented in a social-ecological model framework (numerous individual factors, interpersonal factors, environmental factors). The model posits that the moderating factors influence the likelihood of practicing yoga through mediating mechanisms including practitioners' perceptions of social norms about yoga, self-efficacy to practice yoga, and social support to practice yoga. The authors specifically highlight the goals of interventionists ought to be targeting the mediating mechanisms to increase participation in yoga.

My conceptual model synthesizes and adds to the 2 models mentioned above. I hypothesize that some characteristics may be associated with maintenance of yoga practice through their effect on adoption of any kind of yoga practice generally. Other facilitators/barriers specifically apply to certain modes of yoga practice, specifically instructor-led group practice and independent practice. For example, the social dynamics of a group yoga practice may be associated with maintenance of yoga practice generally, but only through those yoga practitioners who attend group classes with an instructor. Alternatively, some factors that may seem to be barriers to yoga may only be barriers to one mode of delivery. For example, scheduling and logistics may be an important barrier to group practice but not to independent practice. In the model, it is important to consider independent and instructor-delivered yoga modes separately to understand their relative contributions to outcomes.

In the model, a person's baseline attitudes, use of other health practices, personality and pain change the likelihood of practicing yoga. In addition, independent and instructor-led modes of yoga practice each have unique barriers and facilitators. These modes of practice have some unknown relationship with each other. Yoga may lead practitioners to develop new attitudes toward yoga, new use of other health practices, and changes in pain or other biometrics. These new characteristics may lead to maintenance of yoga practice and development of a regular yoga practice.

Figure G-2: Conceptual model of the relationship between modes of yoga practice and maintenance of yoga practice

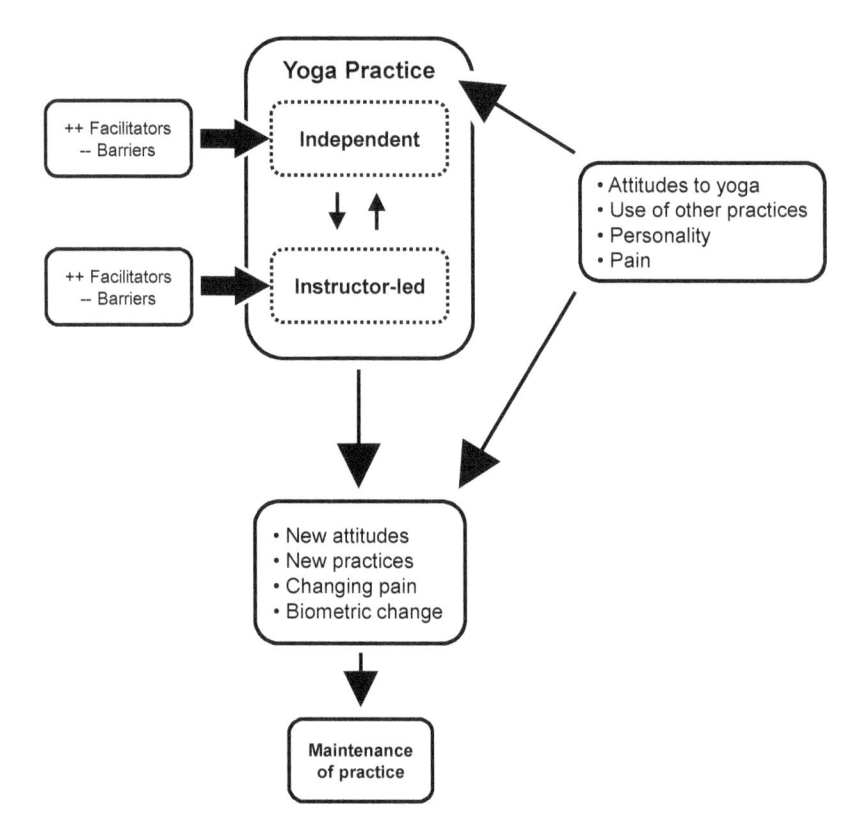

Yoga Practice
- Independent
- Instructor-led

++ Facilitators
-- Barriers

++ Facilitators
-- Barriers

- Attitudes to yoga
- Use of other practices
- Personality
- Pain

- New attitudes
- New practices
- Changing pain
- Biometric change

Maintenance of practice

G.3. Operationalizing resilience and vulnerability coping factors

Table G-1: Proposed pain resilience and vulnerability factors collected as part of the main dataset.

Domain	Construct	Measure
Psychological Distress	Depressive symptoms	PHQ-8
	PTSD symptoms	PCL-5
Pain-related Behaviors	Illicit substance use	DAST-10
	Alcohol use	AUDIT-C
Personality	Absorption	MPQ-BF

Abbreviations
PHQ-8:   Patient Health Questionnaire depression scale[87]
PCL-5:   PTSD Checklist[103]
DAST-10: Drug Abuse Screening Test[90]
AUDIT-C: Alcohol Use Disorders Identification Test[91]
MPQ-BF: Multidimensional Personality Questionnaire Brief Form[104]

G.3.i. *Depressive symptoms*

Depressive symptoms are common among people with chronic pain. Up to half of people with chronic pain experience comorbid depressive symptoms.[105,106] Prevalent depression is a strong predictor of incident chronic pain, and vice versa.[106] Depressive symptoms are associated with higher pain interference.[86] Presence of chronic pain or depressive symptoms appears to negatively influence recognition and diagnosis of the other.[107] These relationships were found to be strengthened among veterans deployed to Iraq or Afghanistan.[108]

The Patient Health Questionnaire-8 (PHQ-8) Depression scale[109] was used to measure depressive symptoms. The PHQ-8 is an 8-item self-report questionnaire that asks respondents to report the frequency they experienced each of the 8 items over the preceding 2 weeks. Each item can be scored 0 to 3 for frequency (0: not at all; 3: nearly every day), which gives a total score range of 0 to 24. A score of 0 to 4 represents no significant depressive symptoms and 20 to 24 represents presence of severe depressive symptoms. The PHQ-8 shows strong internal consistency and test-retest reliability[110,111] and convergence with other depression scale scores[90,112] and self-reported disability days and clinic visits.[113] Figure I-1 (p. 34) shows the 8 items of the PHQ-8.

G.3.ii. *PTSD symptoms*

Post-traumatic stress disorder (PTSD) is an important cause of disability and healthcare utilization in deployment veterans. In fact, it is the most commonly diagnosed mental health condition affecting care-seeking veterans of the recent deployments in Iraq and Afghanistan.[114] PTSD is characterized by an index near-death experience or witnessed near-death experience, intrusive recurrent memories of the event, avoidance behavior and hyperarousal.[115] PTSD is associated with worse clinical pain outcomes[116] and high-risk pain analgesic use.[117] Veterans with chronic pain and comorbid PTSD are more than twice as likely to receive opioids for their pain than those without PTSD[117] and experience more intense and disabling pain than those without PTSD.[108]

Post-traumatic stress symptoms were measured with the PTSD Checklist-5 (PCL-5).[118] The PCL is broadly used and it evidences strong psychometric properties[119,120] and convergent relations with interview assessment of PTSD symptoms.[88,118] The PCL-5 is a 20 question self-report scale that asks respondents to report how much they have been bothered over the past week by the 20 possible problems (0: not at all bothered; 4: extremely bothered). It has a score range of 0 to 80. A cut score of 33 has a 93% sensitivity and 72% specificity for PTSD according to DSM-V criteria.[118] Figure I-2 (p. 35) shows the 20 items of the PCL-5.

G.3.iii.   *Illicit substance use*

Comorbid substance use disorder is associated with worse outcomes in chronic pain including increased interference, decreased function and less pain improvement.[11] Comorbid substance use is more prevalent in veterans than the US adult population[121] and is commonly comorbid with PTSD and depression. Here, illicit substance use is conceptualized as a behavior in response to pain.

The Drug Abuse Screening Test (DAST-10) was developed as a screening tool for substance abuse problems other than alcohol in non-clinical and clinical settings.[90] It has shown sensitivity to illicit substance use in populations ranging from undergraduates,[122] psychiatric outpatients,[123] to individuals with severe and persistent mental disorders.[124] The measure has sound psychometric properties for use with psychiatric outpatients based on criterion-related, concurrent, and discriminant validity.[90,125,126] Figure I-3 (p. 36) shows the items of the DAST-10.

G.3.iv.   *Alcohol use*

Problem alcohol use is common in recent deployment veterans[127] and in comorbid chronic pain but may not be associated with chronic pain,[11,127] although problem alcohol use is more common among veterans with chronic pain and comorbid substance use disorder than without substance use disorder.[92] A history of problem alcohol use is thought to be a risk factor for high-risk analgesic use.[117]

The Alcohol Use Disorders Identification Test (AUDIT)[91] was developed in a cross-national effort by the World Health Organization to identify items distinguishing hazardous from non-hazardous alcohol use. The scale demonstrates strong sensitivity and specificity at a cut-score of 8, with 92% of hazardous drinkers scoring 8 or more and 94% of non-hazardous drinkers scoring less than 8.[128] Figure I-4 (p. 37) shows the items of the AUDIT.

G.3.v. *Absorption*

Absorption is one of 11 personality scales measured by the Multidimensional Personality Questionnaire.[129–131] It is a measure of mindful and open personality. It can be briefly described as the capacity for dedicating one's full attention to the senses and imagination and becoming deeply immersed in those attentional experiences.[130] It is historically tied to complementary medicine because it was originally designed as a predictive measure of response to hypnosis (a complementary modality). Since absorption is positively correlated with openness to experience yet distinct, it is an intriguing personality dimension to study. Openness to experience has been shown to be associated with higher use of and belief in complementary therapies.[132,133] Absorption may predict placebo response.[134,135] Chronic pain patients may be lower in absorption scores than the general population,[136] and higher absorption scores may be associated with somatization.[137] On the other hand, higher absorption may be associated with positive pain coping rather than catastrophizing.[138]

Absorption was measured using the 11-item absorption subscale of the Multidimensional Personality Questionnaire Brief Form.[104] The range of possible scores is 0 to 11, scored by response to 12 yes or no items. Some example items are, "I can be deeply moved by a sunset," and, "Textures—such as wool, sand wood—sometimes remind me of colors or music."

G.3.vi. *Yoga*

Participants were asked to self-report their use of yoga in the previous 12 months. They were asked to respond "Yes" or "No" to the prompt, "In the past year, I have used yoga: practices that combine physical postures, breathing techniques, and meditation or relaxation." Anyone responding "Yes" to past year practice was determined to be in the yoga practice group for this analysis. Participants who reported any past year use of yoga were also asked their past month frequency of practice. The past month frequency options were "Not at all," "Several days," "More than half the days," and "Nearly every day." Also, participants reporting yoga in the past year were asked to report their reasons for practicing yoga. They could report any combination of the three options, "Improve well-being/general health," "Manage pain," or "Manage a condition other than pain." These were not mutually exclusive. [This item comes from the Health Practices Inventory, detailed in Manuscript 3 ("Patterns of non-pharmacological health practices"), and presented in full as Figure L-2 (p. 119)]

H: RESEARCH QUESTIONS AND SIGNIFICANCE

There were several important questions I wished to address with this project. First of all, consistent with the model I have presented, I wanted to know if yoga is associated with a lower prevalence of pain interference ("Cross-sectional association of yoga practice and interfering pain," p.38). I use cross-sectional data from a follow-up study of Minnesota National Guard Veterans to answer this question. The question presents some challenges. Cross-sectionally, yoga practitioners may be in different stages of the time course of their practice and their pain. There will be a mix of new and experienced practitioners so there could be a dilution of mixing of effect. Also, it requires some speculation as to the direction of any effect: does pain interference lead to yoga practice? Do personal factors that lead to improved outcomes in pain also lead to yoga practice? There are likely many effects acting simultaneously. I hypothesize that yoga practice will be associated with a decreased prevalence of pain interference.

Second, I aimed to describe and explain similarities and differences in the yoga practice of those with chronic pain and those without chronic pain ("How pain shapes the experience of yoga," p. 57). If yoga is beneficial in treating chronic pain, does that apply to all yoga practices? If the kind of yoga people use for pain is substantially different from the yoga people use for other reasons, is there a functional reason for that difference? Can yoga practice be distilled into a few key components in order to better study it? I addressed these questions by sending a new follow-up survey to the participants in the first study that indicated they used yoga. I developed and administered a follow-up survey that included personal factors, pain, and a novel implementation of an instrument developed by others to quantitatively describe yoga interventions along a few key dimensions (Essential Properties of Yoga Questionnaire). In addition to the survey, I wanted to talk to yoga practitioners in order to give them the opportunity to further describe their experiences in rich detail. This complex research question required an approach that used multiple types of data and analysis to triangulate towards a deep understanding of pain and yoga. I applied the principles of mixed methods research to use both quantitative and qualitative data to address related but different questions. I took a pragmatic approach to allow the research to be completed in as informative a way as possible given the resources available for the project, and used the qualitative phase to build off of the quantitative phase. I hypothesized that yoga practitioners with chronic pain would be practicing less frequently and using more mindful practices than practitioners without chronic pain.

Third, I was curious about how yoga fits into the larger picture of practices that people use for their health ("Patterns and use of non-pharmacological health practices," p. 90). I expect that yoga practitioners are not using only yoga and may be integrating several practices. Many other practices have been shown to be beneficial for health maintenance and as treatments for various conditions. Understanding the universe of practices that people use in addition to yoga is an important step in teasing apart the benefits of yoga from the benefits of the other practices yoga practitioners use. Also, there may be an organized pattern to how people use practices. It would be beneficial to learn about these patterns and who uses health practices in those ways to better learn how to encourage their use broadly. To this end, I used data from a new checklist of health practices (Health Practices Inventory, p. 119) that was administered during the first study ("Cross-sectional association of yoga practice..."). In fact, this checklist is the way I was able to identify the yoga practitioners in the sample.

I conducted these studies at the Minneapolis Veterans Affairs Medical Center with Minnesota National Guard Veterans. Overall, veterans are a high-need, important population. Their needs and concerns have been and important subject of attention in the media recently. Amidst calls for reform in how medical care is delivered to veterans, providing evidence-based care requires the continuous generation of new evidence. Yoga and other non-pharmacological approaches have strong proponents in the VA and Department of Defense. To inform their efforts to increase use of effective non-pharmacological therapies, I want to shed some light around yoga practitioners who are veterans.

The work presented in this dissertation is important for several additional reasons. I present data from 2 new implementations of useful survey instruments. I have administered a shortened form of the Essential Properties of Yoga Questionnaire to practitioners for the first time. It has previously only been completed by trained expert reviewers to quantitate yoga interventions. This work shows that it can be completed by people who use yoga to describe what they do as a part of yoga, and it picks up on differences in practice that may be otherwise challenging to observe or quantitate by self-report. Also, I have analyzed data from the Health Practices Inventory in order to assess self-reported use of multiple practices. I think it is important to simultaneously consider people's use of multiple practices, and the Health Practices Inventory may facilitate that.

This work has implications in research, clinical care, and population health. Researchers will benefit from the 2 new instruments. Clinicians who provide care to veterans or coordinate pain treatment will benefit from a better understanding of how veterans are using yoga in their pain and what kinds of factors lead them to use yoga. Clinicians will also have a better understanding of the clinically meaningful patterns of use of non-pharmacological practices and how some practices cluster together. These patterns may help clinicians match their patients with effective and palatable treatments. The findings in this dissertation may also inform interventions designed to ease the burden of chronic pain and its comorbidities at a population level. Many non-pharmacological therapies are inexpensive to deliver or use and some have been specifically shown to be cost-effective. Yoga interventions have not always been delivered in pragmatic, realistic ways. This dissertation provides information that may help tailor yoga interventions to veterans or enhance participation in interventions by focusing on key ways that pain affects yoga practice.

The section that follows include an overview ("Study Design," p. 29) of the study population and methods of the survey that provided the data for Manuscript 1 ("Cross-sectional association...") and Manuscript 3 ("Patterns of use..."). The full text of the 3 manuscripts follow in the order presented above. The dissertation ends with a discussion and summary (p. 123), where I unify the findings from the 3 manuscripts and discuss specific implications of the findings.

This dissertation is a beginning and will hopefully facilitate a better understanding of yoga, veteran health, and self-management of health.

I: **STUDY DESIGN**

I.1. Overview of study

The three manuscripts in this study makes use of several different sources of data. This study uses existing longitudinal data collected by the Readiness and Resilience in National Guard Soldiers (RINGS) Project. RINGS-CAM is an NCCIH-funded study that is the latest study to add to the pre-existing RINGS database. First, Manuscript 1 ("Cross-sectional association…," p.38) and Manuscript 3 ("Patterns of use…," p.90) exclusively use data from the RINGS-CAM study (p. 30), a four-year mixed methods study that (as of May 2018) is in the dissemination phase. In RINGS-CAM, 1,850 members of the parent RINGS cohort completed a follow-up survey in 2016 focusing on their current health and utilization of health practices and health services. Manuscript 2 ("How pain shapes the experience of yoga…," p. 57) is a mixed methods investigation embedded within RINGS-CAM (see Figure K-1, p. 80 for schematic). RINGS-CAM participants who reported that they had practiced yoga in the year prior to the RINGS-CAM survey were invited to participate in a follow-up survey focusing on their yoga practice. In addition, a small qualitative interview subsample was recruited from the same eligible participants to explore quantitative findings of the survey in more depth. The follow-up survey data collection and the qualitative interviews were conducted simultaneously. The qualitative interview guide (see Table K-1, p. 81) was designed to cover a wide range of topics that address participants' experiences with yoga. This gave us the flexibility to anticipate potential interesting themes that could emerge in the survey results. The results of the follow-up survey were used as an analytic lens for the qualitative data. The qualitative interviews were also stratified by pain status, as reported in the follow-up survey.

I.2. Description of RINGS-CAM study

The RINGS project is a series of longitudinal cohort studies to identify resilience and vulnerability factors predictive of post-deployment health and health care utilization in soldiers. This work has produced a prospective, longitudinal dataset of 3,458 Army National Guard Soldiers deployed to Iraq and Afghanistan who completed pre-deployment assessments and then followed across multiple waves post-deployment. The *RINGS-1* Study, funded by the Department of Defense, includes Soldiers deployed to Iraq (Operation Iraqi Freedom, OIF) March 2006–July 2007 (n=522) and July 2007–July 2008 (n=229) who completed follow-up waves three months, one year, and two years post-deployment (response rate=81%). The *RINGS-2* Study, funded by VA Health Services Research and Development (HSR&D), includes soldiers deployed to Afghanistan (Operation Enduring Freedom, OEF) July 2010–July 2011 (n=618; response rate=61%) and to Kuwait/Iraq (Operation New Dawn, OND) July 2011–July 2012 (n=2,089) who completed follow-up surveys three months post-deployment. The existing dataset is richly characterized by a set of common data elements, including the following domains: 1) Pre-deployment measures of personality, psychosocial risk/protective factors, baseline mental health symptoms, and pain symptoms; 2) Post-deployment reports of exposure to deployment stressors, mental health symptoms (PTSD, depression, and alcohol abuse), physical health, health care utilization, and pain symptoms; 3) VA administrative data on health services utilization.

The combined RINGS dataset consists of 3,458 Army National Guard soldiers deployed to Iraq who completed pre-deployment assessments and were followed across multiple waves post-deployment. To date, the RINGS data has been used in publications that identified predictors of: PTSD symptom severity, depression, and alcohol abuse[139–142]; occupational status and functioning[143]; intimate partner relationship functioning[144–146]; personality factors associated with health outcomes[140,147]; and barriers/facilitators to treatment-seeking.[148,149]

RINGS-CAM aims to examine chronic pain and use of complementary and integrative therapies (*formerly* CAM, *complementary and alternative medicine*) in the RINGS cohort and to develop a comprehensive model of health services utilization that identifies prospectively assessed predisposing individual characteristics; facilitators and barriers; and need factors predictive of OEF/OIF/OND Veterans' utilization of CAM, other non-pharmacological approaches, and opioid analgesics. RINGS-CAM is a 4-year mixed method study combining data from the existing longitudinal RINGS datasets, new survey data from RINGS participants, data from VA medical records, and qualitative interview data.

RINGS-CAM utilizes an explanatory sequential mixed methods (QUAN→qual) design with the existing sample of Army National Guard Soldiers enrolled in RINGS. In the quantitative phase, participants were administered a battery of valid and reliable self-report questionnaires using standard mailed survey procedures 36-96 months post-deployment. Self-report measures assessed pain intensity and interference, comorbid mental health symptoms (including PTSD, depression, anxiety, and substance abuse), pain-related coping, pain-related attitudes and beliefs, overall health-related-quality of life, and health services utilization. Primary outcomes included chronic pain and self-reported health services utilization, including use or no-use of four broad categories of pain-management approaches (active complementary therapies, practitioner-delivered complementary therapies, active conventional therapies, and opioid analgesics). In addition, administrative data was extracted from VA electronic medical records to assess participants' utilization of VA pharmacological and non-pharmacological health services. Quantitative information from mailed survey responses and administration data will be merged with the existing richly characterized longitudinal dataset.

I.2.i.   *Inclusion criteria.*

RINGS-CAM extended an on-going observational, longitudinal study of post-deployment health among National Guard Soldiers deployed to Iraq and Afghanistan. In order to be eligible to participate in RINGS-CAM, were listed as a member of the RINGS cohort (participants who completed pre-deployment questionnaires as part of an ongoing prospective, longitudinal study who agreed to be contacted for follow-up studies). With the exception of preliminary cognitive testing for the survey battery, recruitment for the current study was restricted to members of the RINGS registry because the aims of RINGS-CAM require pre-deployment assessments of personality and other risk/resilience factors, which are only available within the RINGS cohort.

I.2.ii. *Exclusion criteria.*

Subjects were excluded from study participation if they have not deployed to Iraq or Afghanistan or did not wish to take part in the study.

I.2.iii. *Enrollment procedures.*

Members of the RINGS cohort who have previously completed a pre-deployment survey and at least one post-deployment survey were eligible for enrollment in RINGS-CAM. Prior to beginning study enrollment for RINGS-CAM, all Veterans listed in the RINGS registry were informed about the study through a RINGS study newsletter which provides updates on the ongoing longitudinal study. The newsletter mailing provided the research team with an opportunity to remind potential subjects of their previous participation in the RINGS Project, to build study affiliation, to generate interest in the forthcoming survey wave, and importantly allowed the study team to track bad addresses and update the tracking system with current contact information. Veterans were invited to take part in the follow-up mailed survey by receiving a pre-notification recruitment letter informing them about the opportunity to participate and informing them that a survey packet would be forthcoming. Those service members who did not wish to participate and did not wish to receive a survey packet could opt out by contacting the research team. About 2-3 weeks later, an initial survey packet was sent to all eligible Veterans. The survey packet included an informed consent letter document detailing the study, their rights to withdraw or refuse, and venues for asking any questions. A waiver of documentation of informed consent is approved for survey procedures in the RINGS study protocol. Veterans were able to refuse to take part in this study at any time (i.e., opting-out by calling a toll-free number included in the pre-notification letter or mailing in a blank survey when they receive the follow-up survey packet).

I.3. Measures

Figure I-1: Items of the PHQ-8

In the past two weeks, how often have you been bothered by any of the following problems?	Not at all	Several days	More than half the days	Nearly every day
1. Little interest or pleasure in doing things.	O	O	O	O
2. Feeling down, depressed, or hopeless.	O	O	O	O
3. Trouble falling asleep or staying asleep, or sleeping too much.	O	O	O	O
4. Feeling tired or having little energy.	O	O	O	O
5. Poor appetite or overeating.	O	O	O	O
6. Feeling bad about yourself - or that you are a failure or have let yourself or your family down.	O	O	O	O
7. Trouble concentrating on things, such as reading the newspaper or watching television.	O	O	O	O
8. Moving or speaking so slowly that other people could have noticed? Or the opposite - being so fidgety or restless that you have been moving around a lot more than usual.	O	O	O	O

Figure I-2: PCL-5 20 items

In the past month, how much were you bothered by:	Not at all	A little bit	Moderately	Quite a bit	Extremely
1. Repeated, disturbing, and unwanted memories of the stressful experience?	O	O	O	O	O
2. Repeated, disturbing dreams of the stressful experience?	O	O	O	O	O
3. Suddenly feeling or acting as if the stressful experience were actually happening again (as if you were actually back there reliving it)?	O	O	O	O	O
4. Feeling very upset when something reminded you of the stressful experience?	O	O	O	O	O
5. Having strong physical reactions when something reminded you of the stressful experience (e.g., heart pounding, trouble breathing, sweating)?	O	O	O	O	O
6. Avoiding memories, thoughts, or feelings related to the stressful experience?	O	O	O	O	O
7. Avoiding external reminders of the stressful experience (for example, people, places, conversations, activities, objects or situations)?	O	O	O	O	O
8. Trouble remembering important parts of the stressful experience?	O	O	O	O	O
9. Having strong negative beliefs about yourself, other people, or the world (for example, having thoughts such as: I am bad, there is something seriously wrong with me, no one can be trusted, the world is completely dangerous)?	O	O	O	O	O
10. Blaming yourself or someone else for the stressful experience or what happened after it?	O	O	O	O	O
11. Having strong negative feelings such as fear, horror, anger, guilt, or shame?	O	O	O	O	O
12. Loss of interest in activities that you used to enjoy?	O	O	O	O	O
13. Feeling distant or cut off from other people?	O	O	O	O	O
14. Trouble experiencing positive feelings (for example, being unable to feel happiness or have loving feelings for people close to you)?	O	O	O	O	O
15. Irritable behavior, angry outbursts, or acting aggressively?	O	O	O	O	O
16. Taking too many risks or doing things that could cause you harm?	O	O	O	O	O
17. Being "super-alert" or watchful or on guard?	O	O	O	O	O
18. Feeling jumpy or easily startled?	O	O	O	O	O
19. Having difficulty concentrating?	O	O	O	O	O
20. Trouble falling or staying asleep?	O	O	O	O	O

Figure I-3: DAST-10 items

The following questions concern information about your use of drugs not including alcoholic beverages, during the past 12 months.
"Drug abuse" refers to (1) the use of prescribed or over-the-counter drugs in excess of the directions, and (2) any non-medical use of drugs. The various classes of drugs may include any of those listed above. Remember that the questions do not include alcoholic beverages.

2. Have you used drugs other than those required for medical reasons?
   - ○ No → If no, continue to page 14, question 1.
   - ○ Yes   If yes, continue below.

3. Please answer every question. If you have difficulty with a statement, then choose the response that is mostly right.

a.	Do you abuse more than one drug at a time?	○ Yes	○ No
b.	Are you unable to stop abusing drugs when you want to?	○ Yes	○ No
c.	Have you ever had blackouts or flashbacks as a result of drug use?	○ Yes	○ No
d.	Do you ever feel bad or guilty about your drug use?	○ Yes	○ No
e.	Does your spouse (or parents) ever complain about your involvement with drugs?	○ Yes	○ No
f.	Have you neglected your family because of your use of drugs?	○ Yes	○ No
g.	Have you engaged in illegal activities in order to obtain drugs?	○ Yes	○ No
h.	Have you ever experienced withdrawal symptoms (felt sick) when you stopped taking drugs?	○ Yes	○ No
i.	Have you had medical problems as a result of your drug use (e.g., memory loss, hepatitis, convulsions, bleeding)?	○ Yes	○ No

Figure I-4: Alcohol Use Disorders Identification Test (AUDIT) items

Please describe your use of alcoholic beverages in the past 12 months. Please respond to these questions even if you have not drank alcohol lately. By a "drink," we mean a can or bottle of beer, a glass of wine or wine cooler, a shot of liquor, or a mixed drink with liquor in it.

1. How often do you have a drink containing alcohol?
   ○ Never
   ○ Monthly or less
   ○ 2-4 times a month
   ○ 2-3 times a week
   ○ 4 or more times a week

2. How many drinks containing alcohol do you have on a typical day when you are drinking?
   ○ I don't drink   ○ 5 or 6
   ○ 1 or 2   ○ 7 to 9
   ○ 3 or 4   ○ 10 or more

3. How often do you have 6 or more drinks on one occasion?
   ○ Never
   ○ Less than monthly
   ○ Monthly
   ○ Weekly
   ○ Daily or almost daily

4. How often during the last year have you found that you were not able to stop drinking once you had started?
   ○ Never
   ○ Less than monthly
   ○ Monthly
   ○ Weekly
   ○ Daily or almost daily

5. How often during the last year have you failed to do what was normally expected of you because of drinking?
   ○ Never
   ○ Less than monthly
   ○ Monthly
   ○ Weekly
   ○ Daily or almost daily

6. How often during the last year have you needed a first drink in the morning to get yourself going after a heavy drinking session?
   ○ Never
   ○ Less than monthly
   ○ Monthly
   ○ Weekly
   ○ Daily or almost daily

7. How often during the last year have you had a feeling of guilt or remorse after drinking?
   ○ Never
   ○ Less than monthly
   ○ Monthly
   ○ Weekly
   ○ Daily or almost daily

8. How often during the last year have you been unable to remember what happened the night before because of your drinking?
   ○ Never
   ○ Less than monthly
   ○ Monthly
   ○ Weekly
   ○ Daily or almost daily

9. How often during the last year have you used alcohol to manage pain?
   ○ Never
   ○ Less than monthly
   ○ Monthly
   ○ Weekly
   ○ Daily or almost daily

10. Have you or someone else been injured because of your drinking?
    ○ No
    ○ Yes, but not in the past year
    ○ Yes, during the past year

11. Has a relative, friend, doctor, or other health care worker been concerned about your drinking or suggested you cut down?
    ○ No
    ○ Yes, but not in the past year
    ○ Yes, during the past year

J: MANUSCRIPT 1:

Cross-sectional association of yoga practice and interfering pain

J.1. Introduction

Chronic pain is a leading cause of disability among American adults[150]; however, for the majority of people who experience chronic pain, their pain does not seriously interfere with their daily life.[89] People who experience pain that does not interfere with their daily life have low interference pain. U.S. Veterans experience chronic pain at a higher prevalence than the civilian population,[151] and with high rates of comorbidities, including traumatic brain injuries, post-traumatic stress, and depression.[127,152–154] Approximately half of U.S. Veterans of the recent wars in Iraq and Afghanistan have chronic pain.[155] Thus, pain is a high priority concern in the institutions that provide medical care to veterans and the military.[27]

Yoga is a complementary practice used by many Americans with pain,[156] particularly because of its safety,[157] and the incomplete effectiveness of conventional pharmacological pain treatments.[158] Yoga has been demonstrated to be effective in the treatment of low back pain and is a recommended adjunctive therapy.[79,159–162] Yoga appears to be more common among American adults with painful musculoskeletal conditions than those without pain,[156] but findings are mixed.[48,49] Evidence from randomized trials shows that yoga reduces pain interference among practitioners.[79(p34)]

Yoga practice is associated with higher rates of some risk factors for high pain interference.[48] Depressive symptoms are associated with higher pain interference[86] and may be associated with higher use of yoga.[48] Anxiety appears to be associated with higher pain interference[163,164] and yoga practice.[48] There is unclear evidence on other important risk factors, including PTSD and substance use. Data on the association of pain interference risk factors and yoga practice are quite limited. This is an important gap to explore because these interference risk factors may confound the relationship between yoga practice and pain interference in non-randomized study designs.

The evidence base of yoga for chronic conditions is especially sparse in military and veteran populations.[79,165,166] Veterans and other military personnel may use of complementary therapies at higher rates than civilians;[167] however, veterans may use yoga at lower rates.[165] Additionally, previously conducted randomized interventions of yoga for chronic pain have been conducted with samples that have low rates of pain comorbidities and may not generalize well to veteran populations.[168]

Based on the evidence that yoga reduces pain interference in trials and the association between yoga practice and higher pain interference comorbidities, yoga practitioners may initially begin with higher pain interference that decreases over time; however, yoga practitioners generally report using yoga for their overall health and wellness, not to manage pain.[45,169–171] In a cross-sectional analysis, it is unclear how these factors would balance and if these factors would be observed among veterans who practice yoga.

The main aim of this study was to estimate the association of yoga practice and pain interference, controlling for demographic, deployment experience, substance use, mental health and personality variables that may potentially confound this association. The hypothesis of this analysis is that yoga practitioners will be less likely to report moderate or severe pain interference (versus low pain interference) than non-yoga practitioner controls in this sample. To better understand this association, there were 3 other explanatory aims: 1) estimate bivariate associations of demographic, deployment experience, substance use, mental health and personality variables and pain interference; 2) estimate bivariate associations of demographic, deployment experience, substance use, mental health and personality variables and yoga practice; 3) compare reason for using yoga between the yoga practitioners with high interference pain and the yoga practitioners with low interference pain.

J.2. Methods

J.2.i. *Data Source*

The data for the present study come from the Readiness and Resilience in National Guard Soldiers (RINGS) cohort.[139] Previous studies from the RINGS project have identified pre-deployment resilience and vulnerability factors predictive of post-deployment health and health care utilization in soldiers. 3,890 Army National Guard Soldiers deployed to Iraq, Afghanistan or Kuwait between 2006 and 2011 enrolled in RINGS and completed pre-deployment and multiple waves of post-deployment assessments.

The data for this manuscript come from the most recent follow-up survey (October 2015 to September 2016) administered to members of the RINGS cohort, RINGS-CAM (Complementary and Alternative Medicine). The response rate was 48.2% (n=1,850).

J.2.ii. *Recruitment*

Eligible participants were recruited using a modified Dillman survey procedure 36-96 months post-deployment.[172] Veterans listed in the RINGS registry were informed about RINGS-CAM through a study newsletter, which provides updates on the ongoing longitudinal study. After 2-3 weeks, an initial survey packet was sent to all eligible Veterans. The packet included an informed consent letter detailing the study, their rights to withdraw or refuse, and venues for asking any questions. Veterans could refuse to take part in this study at any time by calling a toll-free number included in the pre-notification letter or returning their survey blank. At 2-week intervals, eligible participants who had not yet responded were mailed a reminder postcard, a second mailed survey, and a final third survey mailed by priority mail.

J.2.iii. *Inclusion/Exclusion*

In order to be eligible to participate in RINGS-CAM, veterans were listed as a member of the RINGS registry, had completed pre-deployment questionnaires as part of the prospective, longitudinal study, and agreed to be contacted for further follow-up studies. All participants were at least 18 years old, served in the Minnesota National Guard, and deployed to Iraq, Afghanistan, or Kuwait between 2006 and 2012. The preliminary cognitive testing for the RINGS-CAM survey was completed with RINGS cohort members who were ineligible because they had not completed pre-deployment questionnaires.

Ethical approval for this study was granted by the Institutional Review Boards of the University of Minnesota and the Minneapolis VA Medical Center. A waiver of documentation of informed consent was approved for this study by both IRBs.

J.2.iv. *Measures*

Respondents were administered a battery of self-report scales assessing pain, comorbid mental health symptoms (including PTSD, depression, anxiety, and substance abuse), overall health-related quality of life, and health services utilization.

Demographics. The main questionnaire covered several broad domains of self-report measures. Participants reported several demographic variables. Age and sex was recorded at time of survey using administrative records. Participants reported their current educational attainment and it was dichotomized at 4-year degree or more versus less than 4-year degree. Participants reported their race. Due to low numbers of participants reporting race other than white, race was dichotomized as white and not white.

Pain. Pain was measured with Version 2.0 of the Graded Chronic Pain Scale (GCPS), which measures self-reported pain severity and interference over the previous 3 months.[173] The scale was scored as indicated and groups were created for no pain (GCPS 0), low interference pain (GCPS I & II) and high interference pain (GCPS III & IV).[173] See Figure J-1 (p. 56) for the 7 items of the GCPS and the scoring rules to define the categories.

Psychological distress. Anxiety was measured on the 8-item PROMIS short form 8a anxiety scale (Patient Reported Outcomes Measurement Information System).[174] Depressive symptoms were measured with the 8-item Patient Health Questionnaire depression scale (PHQ-8).[87] Post-traumatic stress symptoms were measured with the PTSD Checklist-5 (PCL-5).[118]

Substance use. Illicit drug use was measured with the Drug Abuse Screening Test (DAST).[90] The DAST score was dichotomized at 0, above which represents any illicit drug use in the previous year. Alcohol use was measured with the Alcohol Use Disorders Identification Test (AUDIT).[128] The AUDIT score was dichotomized above 7, which represents a cutoff for problem alcohol use.[128]

Deployment experiences. Participants were asked to report if they had participated in combat during any deployment. They could report having directly participated/engaged in combat, observed/witnessed combat but not participated or neither participated nor observed combat. These three options were mutually exclusive. Participants also reported whether they had ever been injured during any deployment. The mechanism of injury and type of injury was also reported. Only the report of injury was used for the present study.

Personality. Absorption (a personality measure of openness to experiences and mindful states), is one of 11 personality scales measured by the Multidimensional Personality Questionnaire.[104,130] Absorption has been shown to be positively associated with use of complementary therapies.[132] Absorption was measured using the Brief Form of the Multidimensional Personality Questionnaire 12-item absorption subscale.[104,130]

Yoga. Participants were asked to self-report their use of yoga in the previous 12 months. They were asked to respond "Yes" or "No" to the prompt, "In the past year, I have used yoga: practices that combine physical postures, breathing techniques, and meditation or relaxation." Anyone responding "Yes" to past year practice was determined to be in the yoga practice group for this analysis. Participants who reported any past year use of yoga were also asked their past month frequency of practice. The past month frequency options were "Not at all," "Several days," "More than half the days," and "Nearly every day." Also, participants reporting yoga in the past year were asked to report their reasons for practicing yoga. They could report any combination of the three options, "Improve well-being/general health," "Manage pain," or "Manage a condition other than pain." These were not mutually exclusive. [This item comes from the Health Practices Inventory, detailed in Manuscript 3 ("Patterns of non-pharmacological health practices"), and presented in full as Figure L-2 (p. 119)]

J.2.v.   *Missing data*

Data on pain was missing for 19 respondents (1%) who were subsequently excluded from all analyses. Further analyses were restricted to this subset (i.e. the 10% of the sample with GCPS 0 were excluded). Of those reporting pain, 16% (n=255) were missing data on at least one measure and were excluded from further analyses. The respondents with any missing items were very similar to those with no missing items (Table J-1, p. 52). Notably, the proportion with any missing items was similar between the high and low pain interference groups (18% [n=64] vs 15% [n=191]) and between the yoga and no yoga groups (15% [n=24] vs 14% [n=210]). The final analysis set was composed of the 1,386 respondents who reported GCPS > 0.

J.2.vi. *Propensity score matching*

Those who self-selected to yoga practice were expected to be quite different from those who did not. Imbalance across a set of confounding factors would introduce bias into an estimation of the association of yoga and pain interference or create a spurious association. Inferences based on participants' self-reported yoga practice could be biased by baseline differences between those who choose to practice yoga and those who do not. Propensity score matching was used to balance potential confounders between exposure groups.[175] Propensity scores allow matching participants on many covariates simultaneously, overcoming the problem of sparseness in high-dimensional matching. A challenge with propensity score matching is that it requires participants in one arm to have a participant in the other arm with a similar score; if there are ranges of the propensity score that do not overlap between the arms, there will be no match, which is called "off-support." This situation can arise when participants in one arm are systematically different from those in the other arm.

Propensity scores model the probability of a participant being exposed (regardless of whether they were or not), conditional on a set of predictors of self-reported yoga practice. Propensity to practice yoga was modeled by logistic regression, entering relevant covariates (sex, absorption, age, educational attainment, mental health comorbidities, substance use, deployment experiences). A predicted probability of having practiced yoga was calculated for each study participant based on the logistic regression and their observed covariates. Each participant was matched (with replacement) to a participant in the opposite exposure arm by propensity score. For example, if a study participant who practiced yoga was calculated to have a predicted probability of practicing yoga (propensity score) of 0.5, they would be matched with the study participant who did not practice yoga who has the closest predicted probability of practicing yoga to 0.5. The analysis proceeded with this matched dataset.

All analyses were performed using the treatment effects estimator of Stata 15.[176] Means or proportions of the relevant covariates were tabulated and stratified by the yoga exposure arms. A propensity score was calculated for each participant, matched participants across yoga exposure arms, and then calculated the prevalence of interfering pain in both arms of the matched sample. Rubin's B and Rubin's R statistics, two measures of balance of covariate means and variances between arms,[177] were calculated using the Stata module PSMATCH2.[178]

The propensity scores showed good overlap between arms and there were no participants who were "off-support." Self-reported general health was excluded from the propensity score because poorer self-report of health is likely caused in part by higher pain interference. Since it is an effect of the main outcome it would not be appropriate to include it in the propensity score model.

The covariates showed good balance after matching (see Table J-4, p. 55). The arms were considered sufficiently balanced based on Rubin's B (20%)

and Rubin's R (0.86) statistics.[177] All matches were within a propensity score caliper of 0.1 and all observations were used.

J.3. Results

J.3.i. *Bivariate associations of pain interference and potential confounders*

Any pain in the past 3 months was reported by 90% of respondents (n=1,641). High interference pain (GCPS III or IV) was reported by 21% of respondents with pain. The subgroup with high interference pain was quite different from the subgroup with low interference pain. Table J-2 (p. 53) presents the bivariate associations between the potential confounders and pain interference. High interference pain was associated with older age, lower educational attainment, having directly engaged in combat during a deployment, having been injured during deployment, worse self-reported health, and higher mental health comorbidities.

J.3.ii. *Bivariate associations of yoga practice and potential confounders*

Any yoga in the past year was reported by 9.9% (n=136) of respondents with pain. Table J-3 (p. 54) presents the bivariate associations of the potential confounders and yoga. Yoga practice was associated with younger age, female sex, higher educational attainment, and higher absorption T-scores. Yoga practice was not associated with the mental health comorbidities.

J.3.iii. *Reason for practicing yoga*

Of those reporting any yoga practice in the past year, 38% (n=51) indicated that they used it for pain. The proportion of those using yoga for pain was higher among those reporting yoga practice at least a few times a month than those reporting less frequent yoga practice (44% versus 31%). Those not reporting using yoga for pain reported using yoga for general well-being (60%, n=82). Yoga users with high interference pain were over twice as likely to report using yoga for pain as were yoga users with low interference pain (67% versus 30%).

J.3.iv. *Multivariable association of yoga practice and pain interference*

Without adjusting for any potential confounders, yoga was not associated with pain interference (unadjusted risk difference=−0.02 [95% CI: −0.09 to 0.06]). In an unmatched analysis, controlling for the same covariates used in the propensity score analysis, yoga practice was not associated with pain interference (risk difference: 0.03 [95% CI: −0.04 to 0.10]). In the propensity score matched analysis, yoga practice was not associated with pain interference (risk difference: 0.03 [95%CI: −0.07 to 0.13]).

Frequency of practice did not influence the association of yoga and pain interference. Of those reporting yoga, 60% (n=81) reported practicing yoga at least several days in the past month. Participants with pain who used yoga in the past month had a similar prevalence of high interference pain compared to participants with pain who used yoga in the past year but not the past month (16% [n=14] versus 21% [n=15]). There was a much higher prevalence of high interference pain among those who used yoga the most frequently, "nearly every day" in the past month (43% [n=6]), but this group was very small and the confidence intervals of the risk difference of the main effect were very large (risk difference: 0.19 [95% CI: −0.051 to 0.43], compared to no yoga in past year).

Yoga practice was also not associated with pain interference when a continuous indicator of practice frequency was used. Participants were not stratified by these finer categories of yoga frequency for the propensity score matching because the groups were too small and past month frequency was missing for an additional 10% of the sample.

J.4. Discussion

In this cross-sectional analysis, there was no evidence of an association between having practiced yoga in the previous year and experiencing high interference pain among a sample of Minnesota National Guard Veterans with pain. The results of the propensity-score matched were similar to the results of logistic regression, which provides additional validation of the results. The yoga practitioners were quite similar to the non-yoga practitioners in the sample, notably among the variables that were associated with high interference pain in the overall sample. In bivariate analysis, high interference pain was associated with worse PTSD symptoms, higher anxiety, more depression, more severe deployment experiences, but these variables were not associated with yoga practice. Only open and mindful personality (absorption) was associated with both high pain interference and yoga practice. In addition, relatively few of the yoga practitioners reported using yoga for pain, although the yoga practitioners who experience high interference pain were much more likely to be using yoga for pain.

These results were unexpected. Yoga practice was associated with demographic variables in the opposite direction as the demographics were associated with high interference pain, yet yoga practice was not associated with lower pain interference. Though the deployment experience variables (deployment injury and combat exposure) had a strong association with pain interference, they were not associated with yoga practice. This could mean having interfering pain does not influence whether someone uses yoga, or it could mean that people who begin yoga with higher interference pain experience a reduction in pain. These different explanations would not be recognizable in this cross-sectional analysis.

In light of high-profile calls for changing what is seen as a historical mismanagement of pain,[14,27,179] accessing non-pharmacological approaches to managing chronic pain in veterans is seen as particularly important.[180–183] Yoga is an intriguing means of improving clinical outcomes for veterans with chronic pain. In randomized trials, yoga interventions have demonstrated significant improvements in short- and long-term pain, pain interference and health-related quality of life.[41,184,185]

There are several limitations in this study. This analysis is based on cross-sectional data so one can only speculate about the causal relationship between yoga practice and pain interference. Propensity score matching is only valid under the assumptions of: 1) no unmeasured confounding; 2) that each participant has a non-zero probability of being treated and untreated; and 3) that the probability of the outcome and treatment of any participant does not affect the probabilities of other participants. The degree to which they are plausible is a limitation. These limitations highlight the importance of validating these findings in independent samples.

This study makes several important contributions. The association of psychological distress and yoga practice is unclear. This study has shown no association between psychological distress and use of yoga among veterans with pain. This study has also demonstrated characteristics of National Guard Veterans who use yoga, which may be of interest to the research and veterans' health communities. The characteristics studied here should be studied in longitudinal designs to better understand the direction of effects. The characteristics should also be studied in prospective designs to explore their role in initiation of yoga.

J.5. Tables and Figures

Table J-1: Comparison of characteristics of sample for complete case analysis compared to those excluded because of missing data

	Complete (N = 1,386)	Any Missing (N = 255)
Age, Mean (SD)	39.1 (9.1)	37.5 (9.5)
Male, % (N)	91% (1,258)	88% (224)
White, % (N)	90% (1,243)	89% (226)
Obtained 4-year degree, % (N)	43% (600)	38% (85)
High interference pain, % (N)	21% (292)	25% (64)
Yoga in past year, % (N)	9.8% (136)	10.3% (24)
Direct Combat experience, % (N)		
None	25% (345)	31% (73)
Observed/witnessed	21% (287)	20% (47)
Engaged/participated	54% (754)	48% (112)
Self-reported general health excellent/very good vs good/fair/poor, % (N)	40% (555)	37% (94)
DAST > 0, % (N)	10% (141)	8.7% (18)
AUDIT score > 7, % (N)	5.3 (5.2)	5.9 (6.4)
PCL score, Mean (SD)	18.0 (17.9)	20.8 (20.0)
PROMIS Anxiety Score, Mean (SD)	15.9 (7.3)	16.3 (7.9)
PHQ-8 score, Mean (SD)	6.0 (5.3)	6.4 (5.8)
MPQ-BF Absorption scale score, Mean (SD)	5.0 (2.9)	4.9 (2.9)

Abbreviations used: DAST, Drug Abuse Screening Test; AUDIT, Alcohol Use Disorders Identification Test; PCL, PTSD Checklist; PROMIS, Patient Reported Outcomes Measurement Information System; PHQ, Patient Health Questionnaire; MPQ-BF, Multidimensional Personality Questionnaire Brief Form

Table J-2: Characteristics of participants with low interference pain compared to high interference pain

Characteristic	High interference (n = 292)	Low interference (n = 1,094)	Difference [95% CI]*
Age, Mean (SE)	41.0 (0.6)	38.6 (0.3)	2.3 [1.2 to 3.5]
Male, % (N)	91% (266)	91% (992)	0.5% [−3.2% to 4.2%]
White, % (N)	85% (249)	91% (994)	−5.8% [−10% to 1.4%]
Obtained 4-year degree, % (N)	34% (98)	46% (502)	−13% [−19% to −6.3%]
Yoga in past year, % (N)	9.3% (27)	10% (109)	−0.8% [−4.6% to 3.0%]
Direct Combat experience, % (N)			
None	17% (49)	27% (296)	<0.0001†
Observed/witnessed	19% (55)	21% (232)	
Engaged/participated	64% (188)	52% (566)	
Injured during a deployment	52% (152)	25% (268)	27% [21% to 34%]
Self-reported general health excellent/very good vs good/fair/poor, % (N)	16% (48)	46% (507)	−30% [−35% to −25%]
DAST > 0, % (N)	12% (36)	9.6% (105)	2.9% [−1.3% to 7.1%]
AUDIT score > 7, % (N)	25% (73)	21% (229)	3.8% [−1.7% to 9.4%]
PCL score, Mean (SE)	33.4 (1.2)	13.9 (0.4)	19.4 [17.4 to 21.5]
PROMIS Anxiety Score, Mean (SE)	21.1 (0.5)	14.5 (0.2)	6.5 [5.6 to 7.4]
PHQ-8 score, Mean (SE)	10.5 (0.3)	4.8 (0.1)	5.7 [5.1 to 6.3]
MPQ-BF Absorption T-score, Mean (SE)	49.3 (0.7)	47.7 (0.3)	1.7 [0.3 to 3.0]

* Absolute differences. Percentages are on the additive scale and are not the relative change.

† Fisher's exact test for trend

Abbreviations used: DAST, Drug Abuse Screening Test; AUDIT, Alcohol Use Disorders Identification Test; PCL, PTSD Checklist; PROMIS, Patient Reported Outcomes Measurement Information System; PHQ, Patient Health Questionnaire; MPQ-BF, Multidimensional Personality Questionnaire Brief Form

Table J-3: Characteristics of yoga practitioners with pain compared to non-yoga practitioners with pain.

	Yoga practitioners (n=136)	Not yoga practitioners (n=1,250)	Difference [95% CI]*
Age, Mean (SE)	36.3 (0.7)	39.4 (0.3)	−3.1 [−4.7 to −1.5]
Male, % (N)	73% (99)	93% (1,159)	−19% [−27% to −12%]
White, % (N)	93% (127)	90% (1,116)	3.6% [−0.9% to 8.1%]
Obtained 4-year degree, % (N)	58% (79)	42% (521)	16% [7.4% to 25%]
High interference pain, % (N)	20% (27)	21% (265)	−1.6% [−8.6% to 5.5%]
Direct Combat experience, % (N)			
None	26% (35)	24% (310)	0.47†
Observed/witnessed	24% (33)	20% (254)	
Engaged/participated	50% (68)	55% (686)	
Injured during a deployment	29% (39)	31% (381)	−2.1% [−10% to 5.9%]
Self-reported general health (%, N) excellent/very good vs good/fair/poor	48% (65)	39% (490)	8.6% [−0.2% to 17%]
DAST > 0, % (N)	15% (21)	9.6% (120)	6.0% [−0.3% to 12%]
AUDIT score > 7, % (N)	27% (37)	21% (265)	5.7% [−2.1 to 14%]
PCL score, Mean (SE)	17.7 (1.3)	18.1 (0.5)	−0.5 [−3.7 to 2.7]
PROMIS Anxiety Score, Mean (SE)	16.7 (0.6)	15.8 (0.2)	0.9 [−0.4 to 2.2]
PHQ-8 score, Mean (SE)	5.9 (0.4)	6.0 (0.2)	−0.2 [−1.1 to 0.8]
Absorption scale T-score, Mean (SE)	51.9 (0.9)	47.6 (0.3)	4.2 [2.4 to 6.1]

* Absolute differences. Percentages are on the additive scale and are not the relative change.

† Fisher's exact test for trend

Abbreviations used: DAST, Drug Abuse Screening Test; AUDIT, Alcohol Use Disorders Identification Test; PCL, PTSD Checklist; PROMIS, Patient Reported Outcomes Measurement Information System; PHQ, Patient Health Questionnaire; MPQ-BF, Multidimensional Personality Questionnaire Brief Form

Table J-4: Balance of covariates after propensity score matching

Covariate	Yoga	No yoga
Age, Mean	36.3	37.2
Male, %	73%	74%
White, %	93%	93%
Obtained 4-year degree, %	58%	56%
Direct Combat experience, %		
None	26%	28%
Observed/witnessed	24%	22%
Engaged/participated	50%	50%
Injured during a deployment, %	29%	32%
DAST > 0, %	15%	16%
AUDIT score > 7, %	27%	29%
PCL-5 score, %	17.7	18.5
PROMIS 8a Anxiety score, Mean	16.7	17.2
PHQ-8 score, Mean	5.9	6.1
Absorption, Mean	6.0	6.4

Abbreviations used: DAST, Drug Abuse Screening Test; AUDIT, Alcohol Use Disorders Identification Test; PCL, PTSD Checklist; PROMIS, Patient Reported Outcomes Measurement Information System; PHQ, Patient Health Questionnaire; MPQ-BF, Multidimensional Personality Questionnaire Brief Form

Figure J-1: 7 items of the Graded Chronic Pain Scale (GCPS) and scoring

Adapted from Table 4 and Appendix Table in Von Korff 2011[173]

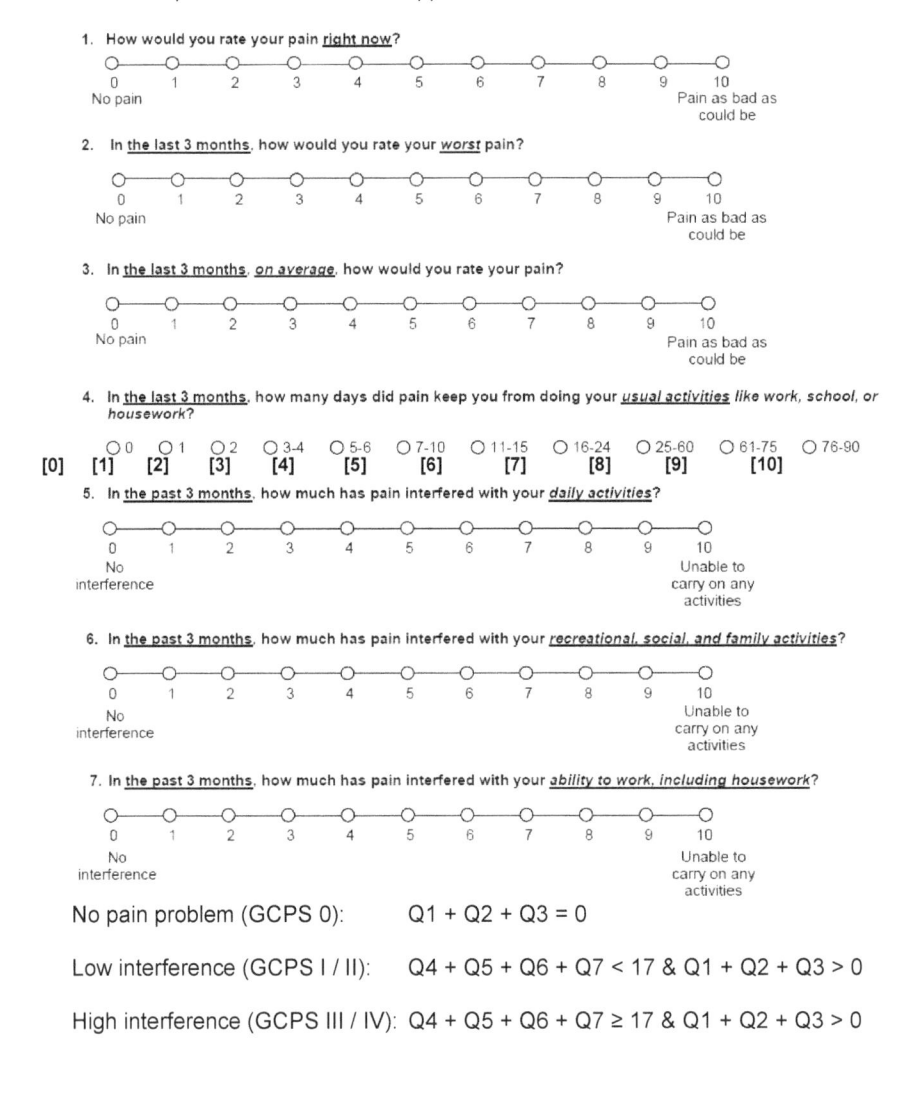

1. How would you rate your pain <u>right now</u>?

   0 — 1 — 2 — 3 — 4 — 5 — 6 — 7 — 8 — 9 — 10
   No pain   Pain as bad as could be

2. In <u>the last 3 months</u>, how would you rate your <u>worst</u> pain?

   0 — 1 — 2 — 3 — 4 — 5 — 6 — 7 — 8 — 9 — 10
   No pain   Pain as bad as could be

3. In <u>the last 3 months</u>, <u>on average</u>, how would you rate your pain?

   0 — 1 — 2 — 3 — 4 — 5 — 6 — 7 — 8 — 9 — 10
   No pain   Pain as bad as could be

4. In <u>the last 3 months</u>, how many days did pain keep you from doing your <u>usual activities</u> like work, school, or housework?

   | 0 | 1 | 2 | 3-4 | 5-6 | 7-10 | 11-15 | 16-24 | 25-60 | 61-75 | 76-90 |
   | [0] | [1] | [2] | [3] | [4] | [5] | [6] | [7] | [8] | [9] | [10] |

5. In <u>the past 3 months</u>, how much has pain interfered with your <u>daily activities</u>?

   0 — 1 — 2 — 3 — 4 — 5 — 6 — 7 — 8 — 9 — 10
   No interference   Unable to carry on any activities

6. In <u>the past 3 months</u>, how much has pain interfered with your <u>recreational, social, and family activities</u>?

   0 — 1 — 2 — 3 — 4 — 5 — 6 — 7 — 8 — 9 — 10
   No interference   Unable to carry on any activities

7. In <u>the past 3 months</u>, how much has pain interfered with your <u>ability to work, including housework</u>?

   0 — 1 — 2 — 3 — 4 — 5 — 6 — 7 — 8 — 9 — 10
   No interference   Unable to carry on any activities

No pain problem (GCPS 0):   Q1 + Q2 + Q3 = 0

Low interference (GCPS I / II):   Q4 + Q5 + Q6 + Q7 < 17 & Q1 + Q2 + Q3 > 0

High interference (GCPS III / IV):   Q4 + Q5 + Q6 + Q7 ≥ 17 & Q1 + Q2 + Q3 > 0

K: **MANUSCRIPT 2:**

How pain shapes the experience of yoga among veterans: A mixed methods study

K.1. Introduction

Yoga is an increasingly common practice among American adults[186,187] and is a recommended therapy for chronic musculoskeletal pain.[159,161,162,188] Yoga appears to be more common among people with chronic pain than among those without.[48,49] Compared to the general US population, yoga practitioners have higher average baseline pain and more medical complaints;[77,78] however, the relationship between yoga and pain is complex. More people use yoga for general well-being than pain specifically,[48,78,169] and pain may be a barrier to yoga practice for some.[100,102,189] It has not been documented if people with chronic pain use similar yoga practices as people without chronic pain. Additionally, yoga has been specifically recommended as a pain therapy for veterans,[162] but yoga is understudied in military and veteran populations.[79,165,166] Veterans may use yoga at lower rates than civilians.[165] Randomized trials of yoga for chronic pain have been conducted with samples that have low rates of pain comorbidities and may not generalize well to veteran populations.[190] It is therefore important to examine the use of yoga by veterans with pain.

Yoga is a comprehensive system of lifestyle guidance that is rooted in the Vedic traditions of India.[50] Contemporary yoga practices are multi-modal, integrating the practice of distinct techniques including relaxation, meditation, stretching and aerobic exercise.[42] There are dozens of yoga styles and lineages,[191] and given this diversity, it is difficult to generalize the experience of yoga practitioners. Moreover, the majority of Americans practice yoga on their own[187] and may not rigorously follow the teachings of any particular style.

There were four main goals in this study: 1) compare characteristics of veterans who practice yoga with and without chronic pain; 2) compare pain between continuing and discontinued veterans who practice yoga; 3) examine differences in yoga practice between those with and without chronic pain; 4) qualitatively explain the main differences in yoga practice between people with and without chronic pain. The final qualitative strand was designed to expand and build upon the findings from the quantitative strand, to gain additional insight into how participants in this study use yoga, and to triangulate the findings from both components.[192] In this sample of young veterans,

K.2. Methods

K.2.i. *Mixed methods overview*

This mixed methods design (QUAN + qual) includes quantitative analysis of survey results of 141 yoga practitioners and qualitative analysis of 11 semi-structured in-depth interviews with yoga practitioners who had chronic pain. Figure K-1 (p. 81) presents the design of this study in schematic form. The quantitative survey phase focused on demographics and pain of practitioners; the context in which they practice yoga, including location, format and length of experience; and the components of their usual yoga practice. This survey includes a pilot of a self-report version of a Brief Form of the Essential Properties of Yoga Questionnaire (EPYQ).[73] The EPYQ, was developed to allow investigators to quantitate their yoga interventions along multiple dimensions. A major goal of the EPYQ is to facilitate comparison of yoga interventions between studies and ultimately allow analysis of the effects of individual components of yoga practices.

For the qualitative phase of the study, 13 interview participants were purposefully selected to obtain diverse perspectives across a range of pain status, age and gender. The interviews followed a semi-structured format that focused broadly the role of pain in the experience of yoga and the role of yoga in the experience of pain among yoga practitioners with pain. The interview included questions on initiation of yoga, perceived benefits of yoga, how participants' yoga practice has changed over time, and participants' thoughts on yoga individually versus with others. Although the interviews were conducted concurrently with the survey phase, analysis of the interviews was conducted after the quantitative analysis was complete to be able follow-up main several findings from the quantitative phase.

The reason for collecting and analyzing both quantitative and qualitative data is to complement the strengths of each approach and to build a richer understanding of variety of experiences of yoga and pain than each approach offers phenomenon on its own.

K.2.ii.   *Participants and Procedures*

This study is nested in a larger mixed methods study of chronic pain and complementary therapy use by veterans, Readiness and Resilience in National Guard Soldiers—Complementary and Alternative Medicine (RINGS-CAM).

National Guard Veterans (n=1850) from a longitudinal cohort responded to a follow-up mailed survey, conducted from October 2015 to September 2016.

Eligibility for the present study was based on a single-item dichotomous indicator of yoga practice, from the Health Practices Inventory (Donaldson et al, in review). Participants in RINGS-CAM, were asked, "In the past year, I have used yoga," and they could respond, "Yes" or "No." A total of 174 respondents from RINGS-CAM reported that they had used yoga in the previous 12 months and were eligible for the present study.

For the present study, data were collected using standard mailed survey methodology.[172] A follow-up questionnaire, cover letter containing all elements of informed consent, and $20 incentive were mailed to 174 eligible participants (1 had an untrackable address and 1 was deceased). A postcard reminder and one additional survey mailing was sent to non-responders at 2 week intervals. Non-responders to the mailings were contacted by phone up to three times. If a non-responder was reached by phone, they were given the option of completing the full survey by phone or receiving a third survey in the mail. The overall response rate was 82% (n=141). Based on administrative records, non-respondents (18% of eligible) were younger (33 versus 37 years old), fewer men (55% male versus 72% male), had a slightly higher prevalence of chronic pain (44% versus 36%) and had lower educational attainment (45% 4-year degree versus 59%), compared to survey respondents.

All study procedures were approved by the institutional review boards of the Minneapolis VA Medical Center and University of Minnesota. A waiver of documentation of informed consent was approved for this study by both IRBs.

K.2.iii.   *Measures*

Yoga. Participants were asked about the frequency of their yoga practice. If participants indicated that they practiced yoga at least once in the past year, they were asked further questions. Participants who did not practice yoga in the previous year were told to skip the remainder of the survey. Those who did practice yoga were asked for how many years in their entire life they have practiced yoga and how often they have practiced in the past month: never, once, a few times, a few times a week, daily or almost daily. Participants were also asked how many months out of the past 12 they practiced yoga even once, and during those months how often they practiced on average. Practitioners often take months-long gaps in their yoga practice and included this frequency question to better gauge regularity of practice over the course of a year.

Demographics. Participants were asked to report demographics to update records with any changes. This included educational attainment, relationship status and National Guard status. Administrative records were used to determine age at time of survey and gender. Records from the prior survey wave were used to determine previous pain status.

Pain. Characteristic pain intensity and interference was measured using the 3-item PEG scale,[193] a self-report of pain intensity and interference over the previous 7 days. The National Pain Strategy population health pain persistence item (5 response version) was used to define chronic pain as the presence of pain on at least half the days in the previous 6 months.[194]

Self-reported health. Overall health was self-reported using the single-item global heath and 1-year prior health questions from the Veterans RAND 12 Item Health Survey.[195,196] Overall health was dichotomized as excellent/very good versus good/fair/poor.

K.2.iv.   *Essential Properties of Yoga Questionnaire (EPYQ) Short Form*

The EPYQ Short Form has 2 parts (see Figure K-2, p. 88).

Part 1 (Context of yoga). The first part of the EPYQ short form consists of 20 questions about the context of respondents' yoga practice, including location of practice, who or what led the practice, with how many other people they practice, and for how long they practice. All questions in this part begin with a common stem, "When you practiced yoga this past year..." The 20 questions are further grouped under 4 common stems: 1) "how often was is at [location]"; 2) how often was your practice led by [who/what]"; 3) "how often were you with [number of other people]"; 4) "how often was it [duration]." For each context item, respondents endorsed how often their yoga practice involved that item, on a 5-point scale: Never, Rarely, Sometimes, Often, or Very often. The items were dichotomized as Never/Rarely versus Sometimes/Often/Very Often.

Respondents who answered that they regularly practice alone (Sometimes/Often/Very Often) were categorized as "regularly practice independently." Respondents who answered that a yoga instructor directed their practice Sometime/Often/Very Often were classified as "regularly practice instructor-led." A summary factor variable was created as Independent / Instructor-led / Both / Neither.

Part 2 (Properties). The second part (properties) consists of 22 questions about components that may be a part of the respondents' yoga practice. These 22 items cover 7 subscales: breathwork, physicality, active postures, mental & emotional awareness, individual attention, spirituality, and meditation & mindfulness. For each of the 22 questions, respondents were asked, "Over the past 6 months, how much did your yoga practice or instruction include..." For each item, respondents answered on a 5-point scale: Not at all, A little bit, Moderate amount, Quite a lot, and Very large amount. Responses were accordingly score 1 (Not at all) to 5 (Very large amount). Respondents were also allowed to select "Don't know" if they could not understand the item. The question stem was worded to include both instructor-led practice and practice independently. Respondents were asked to consider their practice over the previous 6 months.

Missingness. Of the 110 respondents who indicated that they used yoga in the previous year, 94 (85%) completed all 20 items of the EPYQ Part 1 and 98 (89%) completed all 22 items of the EPYQ Part 2. On Part 2, 8 of the respondents who were not fully complete only skipped one or two items and instead put "Don't Know" for those items. Three respondents (3%) skipped the Part 2 entirely. The number of missing responses for each item in Part 2 ranged from 3 to 6, so every Part 2 item has between 104 and 107 respondents.

K.2.v. *Quantitative analysis*

Characteristics of yoga practitioners were tabulated by chronic pain status and a difference and 95% confidence interval was calculated between the two groups. For the EPYQ Part 1, the items were dichotomized as described above, tabulated by chronic pain status, and a difference and 95% confidence interval was calculated between the two groups. A mean score was calculated for each of the 7 subscales of the EPYQ Part 2 (Table K-5, p.85). As a measure of internal consistency, Cronbach's α was calculated for the EPYQ Part 2 overall and for each subscale. To examine the differences in yoga practice between respondents with chronic pain and without chronic pain, means were calculated for each subscale and each item in EPYQ Part 2, stratified by pain status. Means of the 7 subscales were compared by T-test with unequal variances. All survey data was tabulated and analyzed using Stata version 15.[176]

K.2.vi. *Qualitative interviews*

The qualitative stage of this study used a descriptive qualitative design. A total of 11 semi-structured interviews were conducted, each 30–60 minutes long, with participants from the quantitative phase. The purpose of these interviews was to allow the participants to describe their connected experiences of yoga and pain in richer detail than the survey allowed. To be eligible for the qualitative interviews, RINGS-CAM participants reported pain of at least moderate intensity as measured by the 3-month Graded Chronic Pain Scale 2.0 at the previous survey wave (October 2015 to September 2016), and had pain grades II, III, or IV (see Figure J-1, p.56).[173] Participants were compensated $130 for participating in the qualitative interviews. All study procedures were approved by the institutional review boards of the Minneapolis VA Medical Center and University of Minnesota.

A purposeful, heterogeneous sampling approach was used to obtain a range of diverse experiences that included interviews with men and women, chronic pain status, and a range of ages represented in the study. An experienced qualitative interviewer (MD) conducted the interviews face-to-face in a private room or by phone. Interviews were recorded and then transcribed verbatim by a professional transcription agency. The transcripts were reviewed for errors and de-identified. The interview questions that formed the interview guide are shown in Table K-1 (p. 81). The interviews started with general questions about pain, and how the participant manages their pain, and then shifted to focused questions about yoga. The interview transcripts were associated with interviewer field notes that include important details that would not be apparent from the transcript. The semi-structured format was chosen because the question outline increases the comprehensiveness of the data and makes its collection more systematic. The additional openness of the semi-structured format also creates flexibility to allow the interview to remain conversational and context-driven. The interviews were conducted prior to the survey for logistical reasons, so could not directly follow-up on survey responses.

K.2.vii. *Qualitative analysis*

To understand the perspectives of veterans who practice yoga, both their narratives and the language of the narratives were used in detail. The qualitative analytic software NVivo 10 was used to facilitate the coding process.[197] Qualitative analysis followed completion of quantitative analysis so that the qualitative data could explain patterns observed in the quantitative phase.[192] Analysis was led by the first author and guided by a semi-inductive approach, based on the results of the quantitative phase. Analysis proceeded in two cycles.[198] First, during the error checking and de-identification process, all transcripts were read in their entirety. An initial code list was developed using a structural coding approach to identify recurrent themes in the transcripts. During initial qualitative analysis meetings, the themes were discussed. To ensure rigor and validity in the process, the team actively sought alternative interpretation of the data and looked for rich, meaningful details from the transcripts.[199] In the second cycle, pattern coding was used to refine the initial themes into major themes that were relevant to the questions raised in the quantitative phase.[200] During pattern coding, similar codes from the structural coding cycle were grouped into a smaller number of super-codes. The super-codes reduce and summarize the structural codes to facilitate identification of the major themes present in the qualitative data. A content-analytic summary table was then constructed from the codes to make between-case comparisons.[200]

K.3. Results

K.3.i.   *Results from quantitative strand*

Comparison of pain in continuing and discontinued yoga practitioners. Of the 141 participants, 78% (n=110) reported having continued their yoga practice in the previous year, as opposed to the 22% (n=31) that discontinued yoga practice. Table K-2 (p. 82) presents characteristics of the survey participants. The continuing yoga practitioners had similar education attainment compared to those who discontinued yoga (68% with 4-year degree versus 50%, difference=18% [95% CI: --2.4% to 38%]), and similar pain intensity (PEG score mean=2.5 versus 2.7, difference=-0.2 [95% CI: -1.1 to 0.6]), but better self-rated overall health (60% excellent/very good versus 33%, difference=27% [95% CI: 734% to 46%]), and lower prevalence of chronic pain (37% versus 58%, difference = -21% [95% CI: -40% to -1.2%], as measured by 6-month persistence of pain)

The most-frequent yoga group practiced for at least several days per month during 8 out of the past 12 months. Compared to less-frequent yoga practitioners, the most-frequent had similar self-reported overall health (58% excellent/very good versus 62%, difference=-4% [95% CI: -23% to 15%]), similar prevalence of 6-month pain persistence (40% vs 34%, difference=6% [95% CI: -12% to 24%]), but had more intense pain (PEG=2.9 versus 2.1, difference=-0.8 [95%CI: -1.6 to -0.0]).

Characteristics of yoga practitioners with chronic pain. Table K-3 (p. 83) presents the characteristics and frequency of yoga practice of the yoga practitioners with chronic pain compared to those without chronic pain. The two groups looked very similar. Yoga practitioners with chronic pain were slightly older (mean=39 years versus 35, difference=3.9 [95% CI: 0.7 to 7.1]), less likely to still be active in the National Guard (26% versus 44%, difference=-20% [95%CI: -20% to -0.6%]), and with a similar frequency of yoga practice over the past year. The yoga practitioners with chronic pain were much less likely to report being in excellent or very good health compared to yoga practitioners without chronic pain (41% versus 71%, difference=−30% [95% CI: −49% to −11%]).

Differences in practice between yoga practitioners with and without chronic pain. Table K-4 (p. 84) presents the responses to the EPQY Short Form Part 1, including responses in the total sample and responses stratified by chronic pain status (chronic pain versus no chronic pain). Seventy percent of the sample was regularly practicing yoga independently at home. Many of them were using entirely self-directed practices, but half were also regularly using videos, audio recordings or apps. Additionally, half of the sample was practicing yoga with the guidance of a yoga instructor. A similar proportion was practicing yoga at studios as at gyms and exercise facilities. Most yoga practice was about an hour long.

The yoga practice of respondents with chronic pain was similar to those without chronic pain. Notable differences were that respondents with chronic pain practice less at yoga studios than those without chronic pain (18% versus 41%, difference=−23% [95%CI: −40% to −5.5%]) and practice with groups less than those without chronic pain. Respondents without chronic pain also practice longer than an hour at a time more than those with chronic pain.

Table K-5 (p. 85) presents the results of the EPYQ Short Form Part 2, including responses in the total sample and responses stratified by chronic pain status. The internal consistency of the EPYQ Part 2 was excellent, as measured by Cronbach's alpha (α = 0.90). The internal consistency of the 7 subscales ranged from 0.63 to 0.90. There was broad endorsement of the breathwork items, and very little endorsement of the spirituality and individual attention items. The most endorsed item was "holding poses (longer than a few seconds)."

Compared to respondents without chronic pain, the respondents with chronic pain rated "active postures" lower (difference = −0.4 [95% CI: −0.7 to −0.1]) and "individual attention" lower (difference = −0.4 [95% CI: −0.7 to −0.0]).

The findings from the two parts of the EPYQ together suggest that what best differentiates the yoga practice of people with chronic pain from that of practitioners without chronic pain is the use of shorter, gentler, independent practice at home. The 2 key findings from this phase that were further explored qualitatively were: 1) yoga practitioners with chronic pain use more independent practice than those without chronic pain; and 2) yoga practitioners with chronic pain report gentler practice than those without chronic pain.

K.3.ii.   *Results from qualitative strand*

Eleven participants were interviewed. The participants were 6 men and 5 women, ranging in age from 28 to 54 years (mean=39, SD=8). Seven interview participants met the study definition of chronic pain. Four participants primarily practiced yoga with an instructor, five primarily practiced on their own, and two were both regularly practicing with an instructor and on their own. The participant quotes that follow are labelled according to chronic pain status as reported in the survey and whether they primarily practice yoga on their own, with an instructor or regularly do both.

A qualitative follow-up question was created for each of the 2 key findings from the quantitative strand: 1) why do some participants favor independent versus group practice; and 2) what parts of their yoga practice do participants relate to pain? Quotes were grouped into 6 themes (Table K-6, p. 86). The 6 themes were organized by the follow-up question to which each best relates.

K.3.iii. *Why do some participants favor independent versus group practice?*

The first key finding from the quantitative phase that was explored with the interviews was why some participants preferred to practice with a group or at a yoga studio versus at home. Two themes that favored individual practice or home practice were convenience and feeling self-conscious in group practice. One themes that favored a group practice or yoga studio was the group dynamic/social interaction.

Theme 1: Practicing independently is convenient

Participants with and without chronic pain spoke about the convenience of being able to practice yoga on their own and when they needed it. For participants with chronic pain, practicing independently was a way to manage pain as it arises:

> I can kind of use it now if I feel my back hurting; I know more poses to do to loosen it up again. [...] I got to know my body well enough that I can just perform maintenance kind of on the spot. [chronic pain, independent practice]

Independent practice was a convenient way to be able to practice yoga for busy participants:

> I have a mat and I bought some blocks and things like that. And the more I did it, the better I felt. So, I'm like, okay, now I'm just going to

> have to take the time to do that. So, even if it's like 10 minutes. Because I said, gosh, I can't really squeeze in like 45 minutes when I work 12 hours. I just don't want to take another freaking hour, you know, I want to sleep. So, [my instructor] would show me quick 10 minute little ones to help me relax or get me to fall asleep or something like that. [no chronic pain, both independent and instructor-led]

Several participants commented that alternative formats of delivery were also convenient. One participant who uses several different formats said:

> So I do at least one class and then I've got an App thing that's got like a bunch of different classes from beginner to more advanced and they have one that's post-running that I'll do after I use like the elliptical or just a basic stretching or even a little back pain. […] So I can use something like that or a DVD when I can't get to the gym or they don't have a class. [chronic pain, both independent and instructor-led]

Theme 2: Feeling self-conscious in group yoga settings

Interview participants with chronic pain commented on feeling self-conscious in group yoga settings.

> I just went and bought a DVD from [the store] and started doing it at home in the privacy of my own living room, so I didn't really care, you know? You go to a class and you kind of worry about what others think. [chronic pain, independent]

Others commented about being self-conscious because of limitations they experience specifically due to their pain or feeling like a beginner. One participant commented:

> I've found that it's just better to be by myself, be self-aware and do it on my own, rather than in a group setting. Because it almost makes it worse when you're looking over and you see somebody your same age and they can do all this stuff and you're struggling to even put your sock on. [chronic pain, independent]

Participants that felt like beginners thought they would be more comfortable in a class with other beginners or that their concerns were eased after becoming more experienced.

> I would like to do yoga in a group. And I feel like now that I've done a little bit at home, I'd be a little bit better. Like, if there was a beginners' kind of class. Because some people are so good and I would just feel silly, you know, go in the back of the room or something. So, yeah, if it was people on more my level, I would feel comfortable. [chronic pain, independent]

> I look a little more like I belong there. You know there are the yogi people that… I'm just not one of those people, but I try to fit in a little bit. I kind of like to go in the corner instead, but I do feel like I know their moves a little bit more. [chronic pain, instructor-led]

This participant went on to describe how practicing in a group was the only way she felt like she could get past the distractions that are a barrier to practicing:

> [Yoga] is the one group exercise I like—minus sports—being with a group because, again, I'm very competitive, so it helps me get through it. I don't like to do it by myself […] because I know I'm just too distracted and I don't get in the moment when I know I have dirty dishes or something I'm looking at. [chronic pain, instructor-led]

Participants' initial feelings of self-consciousness may be relieved by interacting with a supportive group:

> I've done it in groups and it's been fun. We always think that people are staring at you or looking at you. They don't care what you wear or what you look like or whatever. So, the groups I've gone into have been positive. [no chronic pain, both independent and instructor-led]

Theme 3: The group dynamic is important

For participants who attend group yoga classes, the group dynamic and social interaction are an important part of the experience.

> It's always been a very positive thing for me to go do. I could be having a bad day and I'll feel like, you know what, I might go to a yoga class and just the environment because [...] when I go I feel the support from the other people. [...] So it's kind of the social aspect of it, too, and just talking to people. That's very helpful. [no chronic pain, instructor-led]

> I like [yoga] with a group. I think it adds a whole different dynamic and flow and even just a vibe and feeling to the room. [no chronic pain, instructor-led]

One participant described the group dynamic as creating accountability:

> I couldn't do [yoga] on my own. I mean if [your friends] don't see you, they'll ask where you're at or the instructor will say everybody's in their right spot—because everybody knows that my spot is back there; don't get in my spot. [no chronic pain, instructor-led]

On the other hand, some find the group setting to be distracting. For example, one participant commented:

> Yoga by myself is difficult. [...] But I find the group to be distracting for the mental part ... when you're in a group, it seems like it's harder to focus on your own—there are outside distracters, like other people. [chronic pain, independent]

K.3.iv.   *What parts of their yoga practice do participants relate to pain?*

The second key finding that was explored was how chronic pain shapes yoga practice. Three themes emerged: first, participants developed skills through yoga for coping with pain; second, participants would modify their practice within the limits of their pain either on their own or with the help of an instructor; and third, for a few participants, pain was a main reason for beginning yoga in the first place.

Theme 4: Yoga teaches pain coping skills

Participants expressed a sense that practicing yoga helped them learn how to better deal with pain.

> It empowered me, whereas before I felt like some kind of crippled victim that maybe needed surgery or going to the VA for physical therapy or whatever. Now I really do feel like I have the tools to prepare my body. [chronic pain, independent]

> And I almost felt like just the calming and the breathing maybe helped me cope with [pain] a little bit better. […] I think the more uptight a person is, the more you kind of feel pain. So, when I relax and do that, my body would just feel—my joints felt better and I kind of tended to feel better in general after. [chronic pain, independent]

> I think [yoga] helps to gather your mindset and kind of put yourself in a calm, relaxed place. […] [Pain]'s kind of like a two-year-old. It's easier to manage them if they're in a relaxed, calmed mindset rather than completely worked up and…you know what I mean? […] I think [yoga] kind of forces you into it. It makes you concentrate on your breathing and your overall mindset. I think it makes you more bodily aware. [chronic pain, independent]

Theme 5: Modifying yoga practice within personal limits due to pain

Participants avoided parts of their yoga practice that aggravated their pain. They described this as knowing personal limits or taking it "at your own pace."

> If I do it too much it will, you know, cause a little bit of foot pain and some pains in my elbows, my neck and back a little bit, too. Because there is such a thing as too much, you know… [chronic pain, instructor-led]

> [W]hen I first started, obviously, some of the poses and stretches are hard. If you've never done them, they're going to be difficult. So, that was something definitely when I first started and had the back pain, learning to do some of those new poses and stretches. At first, they would kind of hurt, but with anything, you take it at your own pace and moderation. [no chronic pain, instructor-led]

> I do what my body can do, but I don't ever over-stretch. [...] When my body hurts on some moves, I just don't do them. [no chronic pain, instructor-led]

Some participants with chronic pain find having a trained instructor critical in order to practice "correctly." One participant commented:

> Yoga is a little...yeah, you're in a group but you're also an individual, you're not participating with somebody else, you're being directed. It's also your own pace in a way because you can say well, I've had enough of this particular thing and then do something that's less painful, less hard to do. But it's really important to be coached. Because you can get a videotape or rather a DVD on yoga and sit in your living room and try and do that but you have no idea if you're doing it correctly... [chronic pain, both independent and instructor-led]

Another participant made a distinction between experience with a knowledgeable instructor versus experiences with less-knowledgeable instructors:

> The class that I did at the VA, because they were directing at, "okay, you have back pain, this is how we're going to manage it." But the classes that are offered in the community, they don't have ones that are like that. It's more like yoga for beginners, yoga for advanced people, you know what I mean? They usually give you alternate things to do but it's really, really difficult to be in a class when you don't know if you're going to be able to do it for two minutes or 30 minutes. [chronic pain, independent]

Others felt able to modify on their own. One participant such participant said:

> I have to put maybe extra padding like an extra towel or something under that knee if I have to go into a pose where you're on your hands and knees. [...] But it really hasn't been very hard. I watch the video and I do it how I can do it. [chronic pain, independent]

Theme 6: Pain is a reason for starting yoga

Several participants identified their pain as the main reason they began their yoga practice.

> I've tried massages, but they tend to get a little bit expensive after a while. I'd go like maybe once or twice a month and stuff. And it obviously feels good, but it wasn't—I could keep getting a massage like every day because I'm like, "oh, okay, now my back still hurts." But I can't keep going in and getting a massage or whatever. So, I took a yoga class... [no chronic pain, both independent and instructor-led]
>
> One of my doctors—and I don't remember which one—suggested that I go to [yoga]. [...] I think it was mental health that referred me to that. [chronic pain, independent]

K.4. Discussion

This study had several key findings. First, continuing yoga practitioners report similar pain levels as discontinued yoga practitioners, but the continuing practitioners have a lower prevalence of chronic pain and better self-rated health. Among those continuing yoga, the most-frequent practitioners have worse pain than those who practice less-frequently. Additionally, practitioners with chronic pain were using less-physical yoga practice and were practicing independently more often than practitioners without chronic pain. Otherwise, the yoga practice of those with chronic pain looked very similar to those without chronic pain. Key findings from the qualitative strand suggest that: 1) yoga practitioners with chronic pain feel self-conscious in group yoga settings; and 2) practitioners with chronic pain regularly modify their yoga practice within limits they face due to pain.

Independent practice is used by participants of this study (who are all veterans of recent international military deployments) at a high rate, similar to the

US civilian adult population.[187] Those who practiced yoga with instructors often saw the instructors as a very important part of their practice, but there were important barriers identified to practicing with a group and an instructor. Notably, practitioners' feelings of self-consciousness in group yoga settings stemmed from a variety of sources, including body image, feeling like a beginner among experts, and feeling physically impaired. Broadly these can be seen as a barrier to engagement with group practices.

Camaraderie and good experiences with an instructor are facilitators of instructor-led group practice. These factors are similar to findings with participants in a randomized yoga trial,[100] which found relationships with teachers and classmates to be facilitators of yoga class attendance. The authors also found that there is a motivation barrier to home practice,[100] though participants were still very engaged with home practice in the trial.[101] This is important because the participants of the present study are quite different from those of the randomized trial. In the present study, participants were younger, more men, mostly white, had higher educational attainment, come from a different region of the country, and were exclusively military veterans. Studying this motivation barrier, the camaraderie facilitator, and other barriers/facilitators could be broadly applicable. Much of the evidence base of yoga derives from instructor-delivered group practices; however, most people are using yoga at home, by themselves, so research should also focus on the effectiveness of yoga in alternative delivery formats.[201] Guidelines and for yoga intervention trials and recommendations for research encourage researchers to consider home practice as a part of the total dose of yoga.[55,202] Researchers should also consider the ways that home practice may be a different yoga experience or teach different skills and whether this is important. The self-report questionnaire presented here could facilitate such work.

This is the first implementation of the Essential Properties of Yoga Questionnaire as a self-report measure of yoga practice styles. The seven domains of the EPYQ that are represented in the Short Form demonstrated high correlations between what students reported and what expert raters reported,[73] so it may be reasonable to use a self-report. All items had high rates of completion. There is now an instrument available to trained raters to score observed practices and an instrument available for practitioners to self-report on their own practices. There is broad general interest in allowing practitioners to self-report rather than relying on expert raters. Our implementation shows this is feasible. Further psychometric testing should be conducted to validate the questionnaire in a self-report format, and to validate the shortened form.

This study had important strengths. This study successfully piloted a self-report measure of yoga practice that may be used in other contexts. In addition, the responses from the EPYQ were a useful guide to explore qualitative experiences of a sample of veterans with pain who use yoga. Yoga and pain are both clearly complex experiences that require rich methodologies that consider a range of experiences. Additionally, had the analysis been limited to just quantitative measures, important perspectives would have been missed that the qualitative stream identified. Using the two mixed streams in this way allowed a deeper understanding of this important subject.

This study has several limitations. First of all, these data are based on retrospective recall of past yoga practice. Participants might not accurately recall their practice over the course of 6 months or a year and more recent experiences may bias recall. This sample is very different from all yoga practitioners on the whole. The survey results may not be broadly generalizable. The relatively small sample size limited hypothesis testing as only large effect sizes would be detectable. Additionally, the qualitative analysis was very focused with a small number of participants for logistical reasons. The experiences of these participants might not be transferable to others.

These findings have important implications. Population health researchers and interventionists can use self-report from their participants to assess what yoga practitioners use in their practice. Understanding what components certain yoga practitioners use will allow for research into relative effectiveness of components, intervention refinement, and better understanding of yoga "dosing." Additionally, this deeper understanding of yoga can allow matching yoga styles and refinements to specific conditions or potential yoga practitioner needs. If yoga is to be made more available, it will be important to make different kinds of practice available to allow it to be interesting and accessible to diverse practitioners. Interventions should be accessible to the people who could benefit most from them.

K.5. Tables and Figures

Figure K-1: Mixed methods design schematic of this study

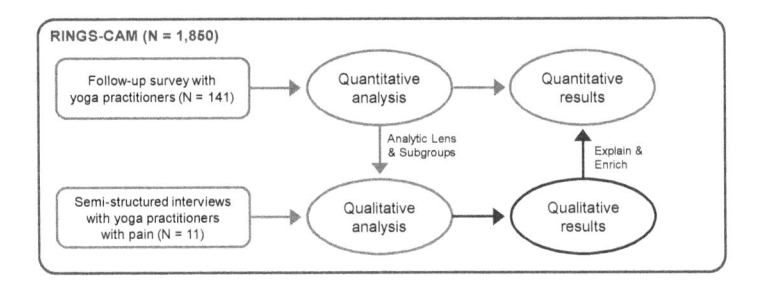

Table K-1: Semi-structured interview guide

1. For background, could you tell me about how your problems with pain started?
    • *How long ago was that?*
    • *How has your pain changed in the last year, if at all?*
    • *How satisfied are you with your current pain management strategy?*

2. Since your pain first started, what kinds of things have you used or tried for your pain? [CLARIFICATION, IF NEEDED: *Such as things you've done yourself to manage pain or different treatments you've tried.*]
    • Why did you start / what drew you to this? [*What made you think it might be helpful?*]
    • Are you still doing it? [IF YES: Why did you stick with it? IF NO: Why did you stop?]
    • What are/were challenges to keeping up with it? Tell me more...
    • Anything else? [REPEAT UNTIL NO ADDITIONAL METHODS]

3. In your personal experience, what has worked best for your pain? Can you tell me more about how [SUCCESSFUL APPROACH] has been helpful? *What do you think is particularly helpful about it?*

4. Have you ever practiced yoga regularly (a few times a month or more)? [IF NO, THEN DISCONTINUE]
    • [IF YES:] Tell me about it.
        ○ How did you get started with that? What led you to start? How often do you practice now?
        ○ Could you tell me about how yoga has or has not been helpful for pain? Why do you think it helped/didn't help? [IF IT DIDN'T HELP: Did it help with anything other than pain?]
    • Could you tell me about how pain has related to your yoga practice (*if it has*)? *Have you adapted/modified your yoga practice because of your pain?* **Has yoga changed your pain or how you cope with pain?** *How so?*
    • Have you talked about pain in yoga class or with an instructor? [IF YES:] How has pain come up in conversation? Have you received or given advice about pain and yoga?
    • Can you tell me about any other ways yoga has affected you personally? *In terms of your health? Your mood? How you think about things?*
    • Tell me about how your yoga practice has changed over time. *In terms of how or when you practice or importance of yoga in daily life.* **Have you had times when yoga has been more or less helpful for you than usual?** *Tell me about that.*
    • What are your thoughts on yoga with a group versus yoga on your own? *How do you feel about yoga as a social activity?*

5. That was my last question. Is there anything that popped into your head as we were talking? Any topics you want to go back to?   • Anything else we should know?

Table K-2: Characteristics of survey participants

Characteristic	Used yoga in past year N = 110 (78%)	Did not use yoga past year N = 31 (22%)
Age, Mean (SE)	37 (0.8)	37 (1.3)
Male, % (N)	69% (76)	84% (26)
Survey conducted by phone, % (N)	7% (8)	13% (4)
Currently under orders from National Guard, % (N)	37% (39)	37% (11)
Currently in school, % (N)	22% (23)	17% (5)
Obtained 4 year degree, % (N)	68% (71)	50% (15)
Relationship Status, % (N)		
Single, never married	15% (16)	10% (3)
Married	76% (80)	87% (26)
Living with partner, not married	6% (6)	3% (1)
In relationship, not living together	3% (3)	0% (0)
Chronic Pain, % (N)	37% (41)	58% (18)
PEG, Mean (SE)	2.5 (0.2)	2.7 (0.4)
Overall health Excellent/Very good, % (N)	60% (63)	33% (10)
Years of yoga, % (N)		
Less than 2 years	25% (27)	--
Less than 5 years but longer than 2 years	43% (47)	--
Less than 10 years but longer than 5 years	22% (24)	--
Longer than 10 years	11% (12)	--
Months of yoga last year, Mean (SE)	7.7 (0.4)	--
Yoga frequency last month, % (N)		
Not at all	33% (36)	--
About once last month	23% (25)	--
A few times last month	25% (28)	--
A few times a week	15% (17)	--
Daily or almost daily	4% (4)	--

Table K-3: Characteristics of yoga practitioners with chronic pain compared to yoga practitioners without chronic pain

Characteristic	Chronic Pain N = 41 (37%)	No Chronic Pain N = 69 (63%)	Difference [95% CI]
Age, Mean (SD)	39.1 (10.2)	35.3 (6.7)	3.9 [0.7 to 7.1]
Male, % (N)	71% (29)	68% (47)	2.6% [−15% to 20%]
Currently under orders from National Guard, % (N)	26% (10)	44% (29)	−20% [−20% to −0.6%]
Currently in school, % (N)	18% (7)	16% (10)	2.3% [−13% to 17%]
Obtained 4 year degree, % (N)	64% (25)	70% (46)	−5.6% [−24% to 13%]
Relationship Status, % (N)			
Single, never married	13% (5)	17% (11)	0.31†
Married	85% (33)	71% (47)	
Living with partner, not married	3% (1)	8% (5)	
In relationship, not living together	0	5% (3)	
PEG, Mean (SD)	4.1 (2.0)	1.5 (1.6)	2.7 [2.0 to 3.3]
Overall health Excellent/Very good,* % (N)	41% (16)	71% (47)	−30% [−49% to −11%]
Years of yoga, % (N)			
Less than 2 years	27% (11)	23% (16)	0.63†
Less than 5 years but longer than 2 years	41% (17)	43% (30)	
Less than 10 years but longer than 5 years	17% (7)	25% (17)	
Longer than 10 years	15% (6)	9% (6)	
Months of yoga last year, Mean (SD)	7.8 (4.3)	7.6 (4.0)	0.3 [−1.3 to 1.9]
Yoga frequency last month, % (N)			
Not at all	29% (12)	35% (24)	0.50†
About once last month	17% (7)	26% (18)	
A few times last month	27% (11)	25% (17)	
A few times a week	22% (9)	12% (8)	
Daily or almost daily	5% (2)	3% (3)	

*Excellent or Very good health versus Good/Fair/Poor health

†Fisher's exact test for trend

Table K-4: Responses to the Essential Properties of Yoga Questionnaire Short Form Part 1

EPYQ Short Form Part 1: Context Item	Total sample N = 110 (100%)	Chronic Pain N = 41 (37%)	No Chronic Pain N = 69 (63%)	Difference [95% CI]
How often at: % (N)				
A yoga studio or other yoga center	33% (33)	18% (7)	41% (26)	−23% [−40% to −5.5%]
Gym, exercise facility or recreation center	47% (47)	42% (16)	49% (31)	−7.1% [−27% to 13%]
Residence or home	70% (76)	74% (29)	68% (47)	2.2% [−6.3% to 11%]
Outside, in nature or at a park	19% (19)	16% (6)	21% (13)	6.2% [−11% to 24%]
How often led by: % (N)				
A yoga instructor, in person	52% (53)	38% (15)	61% (39)	−22% [−42% to 3.1%]
Someone other than a yoga instructor, in person	11% (11)	16% (6)	8% (5)	8.0% [−5.4% to 21%]
A video or audio recording	50% (53)	47% (18)	52% (35)	−4.9% [−25% to 15%]
A book / booklet / pamphlet	9% (9)	11% (4)	8% (5)	2.6% [−9.2% to 14%]
An app	17% (18)	21% (8)	15% (10)	5.7% [−10% to 21%]
Self-directed (from memory or other)	40% (41)	47% (18)	36% (23)	11% [−8.3% to 31%]
How often with: % (N)				
Many other people (20+)	13% (13)	5% (2)	17% (11)	−12% [−34% to −0.0%]
More than a few other people (8-20 other people)	37% (38)	28% (11)	42% (27)	−14% [−33% to 4.6%]
A few other people (2-8)	34% (35)	24% (9)	41% (26)	−17% [−35% to 1.2%]
One other person	29% (30)	21% (8)	34% (22)	−13% [−31% to 4.1%]
Alone / by yourself	71% (75)	77% (30)	67% (45)	9.8% [−7.6% to 27%]
How often: % (N)				
One hour or longer	43% (43)	26% (10)	52% (33)	−26% [−45% to −7.4%]
At least 30 minutes, but less than 1 hour	66% (69)	65% (26)	66% (43)	−1.2% [−20% to 18%]
At least 10 minutes, but less than 30 minutes	49% (51)	53% (20)	47% (31)	5.7% [−14% to 26%]
Less than 10 minutes	22% (22)	24% (9)	21% (13)	3.0% [−14% to 20%]

Study participants were asked to recall their yoga practice over the past 6 months when answering these questions. Percentages are the proportion of respondents endorsing Very Often/Often versus Sometimes/Rarely/Never. The first column is the results of the total sample, then results are stratified by chronic pain status. The final column presents the absolute differences (additive scale) between the chronic pain and non-chronic pain strata.

Table K-5: Responses to the Essential Properties of Yoga Questionnaire Short Form Part 2.

	Total sample	Chronic Pain	No Chronic Pain	P*
EPYQ Short Form Part 2: Properties (α = 0.90) Mean (SD)	N = 110 (100%)	N = 41 (37%)	N = 69 (63%)	
Breathwork (α = 0.83)	**3.7 (1.1)**	**3.7 (0.9)**	**3.6 (1.0)**	**0.69**
Placing one's focus on the breath	3.8 (1.1)	3.8 (1.0)	3.7 (1.2)	
Deep breathing (full inhalation and exhalation)	3.7 (1.1)	3.8 (1.0)	3.6 (1.2)	
Linking breathing with movement	3.6 (1.0)	3.6 (1.0)	3.6 (1.2)	
Physicality (α = 0.83)	**3.0 (0.9)**	**2.8 (0.8)**	**3.1 (0.9)**	**0.08**
Vigorous activity or physical exertion	2.6 (1.1)	2.4 (1.0)	2.6 (1.2)	
Challenging one's physical balance	3.1 (1.1)	2.9 (1.0)	3.3 (1.1)	
Challenging one's physical flexibility	3.4 (1.0)	3.3 (1.1)	3.6 (1.0)	
Challenging one's physical strength	2.9 (1.1)	2.7 (1.0)	2.9 (1.2)	
Active Postures (*Asana*) (α = 0.60)	**3.1 (0.8)**	**2.9 (0.9)**	**3.3 (0.7)**	**0.01**
Modifications to increase the difficulty of a pose	2.9 (1.1)	2.6 (1.1)	3.1 (1.1)	
Holding poses (longer than a few seconds)	3.8 (1.0)	3.5 (1.1)	4.0 (0.8)	
Inverted poses (poses where the head is below the heart or hips)	2.7 (1.1)	2.5 (1.0)	2.9 (1.1)	
Mental & Emotional Awareness / Release (α = 0.90)	**2.8 (1.2)**	**2.8 (1.3)**	**2.8 (1.1)**	**0.82**
Allowing or being present to emotions or feelings that come up while doing yoga	2.4 (1.3)	2.4 (1.5)	2.4 (1.2)	
Mental relaxation	3.3 (1.3)	3.3 (1.3)	3.3 (1.3)	
Emotional release	2.6 (1.5)	2.6 (1.5)	2.7 (1.3)	
Individual Attention (α = 0.63)	**1.7 (0.9)**	**1.5 (0.6)**	**1.9 (1.1)**	**0.03**
Giving individual attention or feedback (instructor or assistants)	1.9 (1.2)	1.7 (1.1)	2.0 (1.3)	
Physically assisting students with poses	1.6 (1.0)	1.3 (0.5)	1.8 (1.1)	
Spirituality (α = 0.78)	**1.5 (0.7)**	**1.5 (0.8)**	**1.5 (0.7)**	**0.85**
Chanting and/or reciting mantras or saying "OM"	1.3 (0.7)	1.2 (0.6)	1.4 (0.8)	
Spiritual readings, quotes, sayings, teachings, or ideas	1.5 (0.8)	1.5 (0.9)	1.5 (0.8)	
Reference to a connection to a higher power or something greater than oneself (Spirit, God, Universe)	1.7 (1.0)	1.8 (1.2)	1.6 (0.9)	
Meditation & Mindfulness (α = 0.87)	**2.4 (1.1)**	**2.3 (0.9)**	**2.4 (1.1)**	**0.52**
Quieting the mind	3.0 (1.2)	3.0 (1.2)	3.0 (1.2)	
Meditation (*Dhyana*: deep absorptive meditation)	2.1 (1.3)	2.1 (1.3)	2.2 (1.3)	
Withdrawal of the senses (*Pratyahara*: directing the attention from the external toward an internal awareness)	2.0 (1.3)	2.0 (1.3)	2.1 (1.4)	
Concentration (*Dharana*: a state of complete absorption or concentration/focus of the mind)	2.4 (1.3)	2.4 (1.3)	2.3 (1.2)	

* P-value of T-test of equality of means with degrees of freedom corrected for unequal variances

Table K-6: Emergent themes (6) from the qualitative analysis that explore 2 key findings from the quantitative phase

Key finding:	Yoga practitioners with chronic pain use more independent practice than those without chronic pain
Follow-up:	*Why do some participants favor independent versus group practice?*

Theme 1: Practicing independently is convenient

- "I can kind of use it now if I feel my back hurting; I know more poses to do to loosen it up again. I got to know my body well enough that I can just perform maintenance kind of on the spot."

Theme 2: Feeling self-conscious in group yoga settings

- "I've found that it's just better to be by myself, be self-aware and do it on my own, rather than in a group setting. Because it almost makes it worse when you're looking over and you see somebody your same age and they can do all this stuff and you're struggling to even put your sock on."

Theme 3: The group dynamic is important

- "It's always been a very positive thing for me to go do. I could be having a bad day and I'll feel like, you know what, I might go to a yoga class and just the environment because when I go I feel the support from the other people."

Key finding:	Yoga practitioners with chronic pain report gentler practice than those without chronic pain
Follow-up:	*What parts of their yoga practice do participants relate to pain?*

Theme 4: Yoga teaches pain coping skills

- "It empowered me, whereas before I felt like some kind of crippled victim that maybe needed surgery or going to the VA for physical therapy or whatever. Now I really do feel like I have the tools to prepare my body."

Theme 5: Modifying yoga practice within personal limits due to pain

- "I do what my body can do, but I don't ever over-stretch. When my body hurts on some moves, I just don't do them."

Theme 6: Pain is a reason for starting yoga

- "I could keep getting a massage like every day because I'm like, 'Oh, okay, now my back still hurts.' But I can't keep going in and getting a massage or whatever. So, I took a yoga class."

Table K-7: Characteristics of interview participants

Characteristic	Qualitative Interview participants (N = 11)
Age, Mean (SD)	39 (8)
Male, % (N)	55% (6)
Currently under orders from National Guard, % (N)	27% (3)
Currently in school, % (N)	9% (1)
Obtained 4 year degree, % (N)	100% (11)
Relationship Status, % (N)	
Single, not partnered	36% (4)
Married	45% (5)
Living with partner	18% (2)
In relationship, not living together	0% (0)
Chronic Pain, % (N)	64% (7)
Years of yoga, % (N)	
Less than 2 years	45% (5)
Less than 5 years but longer than 2 years	36% (4)
Less than 10 years but longer than 5 years	0
Longer than 10 years	18% (2)
Months of yoga last year, Mean (SD)	11 (2)
Yoga frequency last month, % (N)	
Not at all	9% (1)
About once last month	18% (2)
A few times last month	9% (1)
A few times a week	55% (6)
Daily or almost daily	9% (1)

Figure K-2: Full Text of the Essential Properties of Yoga Questionnaire Short Form

YOUR EXPERIENCE WITH YOGA

If you practiced yoga in the past year, please answer the following questions.

The next questions ask you about your yoga practice over the past year. We realize that your yoga practice may have varied over the past year. Try to think about all the times you did yoga over the past year when you answer these questions.

1. When you practiced yoga this past year, how often was it at...

	Very Often	Often	Sometimes	Rarely	Never
a. A yoga studio or other yoga center	○	○	○	○	○
b. Gym, exercise facility or recreation center	○	○	○	○	○
c. Hospital or clinic	○	○	○	○	○
d. Residence or home	○	○	○	○	○
e. Outside, in nature or at a park	○	○	○	○	○

2. When you practiced yoga this past year, how often was your practice led by...

	Very Often	Often	Sometimes	Rarely	Never
a. A yoga instructor, in person	○	○	○	○	○
b. Someone other than a yoga instructor, in person	○	○	○	○	○
c. A video or audio recording	○	○	○	○	○
d. A book / booklet / pamphlet	○	○	○	○	○
e. An app	○	○	○	○	○
f. Self-directed (from memory or other)	○	○	○	○	○

3. When you practiced yoga this past year, how often were you...

	Very Often	Often	Sometimes	Rarely	Never
a. By yourself / alone	○	○	○	○	○
b. With one other person	○	○	○	○	○
c. With a few other people (3-5 other people)	○	○	○	○	○
d. With more than a few other people (8 - 20)	○	○	○	○	○
e. With many other people (20 or more)	○	○	○	○	○

4. When you practiced yoga this past year, how often was it...

	Very Often	Often	Sometimes	Rarely	Never
a. One hour or longer	○	○	○	○	○
b. At least 30 minutes but less than 1 hour	○	○	○	○	○
c. At least 10 minutes, but less than 30 minutes	○	○	○	○	○
d. Less than 10 minutes	○	○	○	○	○

YOUR EXPERIENCE WITH YOGA, continued

Below is a list of some things that can be a part of yoga practice. Think about all the times and ways you practiced yoga over the PAST 6 MONTHS when you answer these questions.

Over the PAST 6 MONTHS, how much did your yoga practice or instruction include...	Very Large Amount	Quite a Lot	Moderate Amount	A Little Bit	Not At All	Don't Know
1. Placing one's focus on the breath?	O	O	O	O	O	☐
2. Deep breathing (full inhalation and exhalation)?	O	O	O	O	O	☐
3. Linking breathing with movement?	O	O	O	O	O	☐
4. Vigorous activity or physical exertion?	O	O	O	O	O	☐
5. Challenging one's physical balance ("finding one's edge" in regards to physical balance?)	O	O	O	O	O	☐
6. Challenging one's physical flexibility ("finding one's edge" in regards to physical flexibility)?	O	O	O	O	O	☐
7. Challenging one's physical strength ("finding one's edge" in regards to physical strength)?	O	O	O	O	O	☐
8. Modifications to increase the difficulty of a pose?	O	O	O	O	O	☐
9. Holding poses (longer than a few seconds)?	O	O	O	O	O	☐
10. Inverted poses (poses where the head is below the heart or hips)?	O	O	O	O	O	☐
11. Allowing or being present to emotions and feelings that come up while doing yoga?	O	O	O	O	O	☐
12. Mental relaxation ("letting go" of mental tensions, worries, or mental stress?	O	O	O	O	O	☐
13. Emotional release ("letting go" of emotions)?	O	O	O	O	O	☐
14. Giving individual attention or feedback?	O	O	O	O	O	☐
15. Physically assisting students with poses (aligning, pressing or stretching a student in a pose)?	O	O	O	O	O	☐
16. Chanting and/or reciting mantras or saying "OM"?	O	O	O	O	O	☐
17. Spiritual readings, quotes, sayings, teachings, or ideas?	O	O	O	O	O	☐
18. A connection to a higher power or something greater than yourself (Spirit, God, Universe)?	O	O	O	O	O	☐
19. Quieting the mind?	O	O	O	O	O	☐
20. Meditation (also called *Dhyana*, or deep absorptive meditation)?	O	O	O	O	O	☐
21. Withdrawal of the senses (also called *Pratyahara*, or directing the attention away from the external toward an internal awareness)?	O	O	O	O	O	☐
22. Concentration (also called *Dharana*, or a state of complete absorption/concentration/focus of the mind)?	O	O	O	O	O	☐

L: MANUSCRIPT 3:

Patterns of use of non-pharmacological health practices

L.1. Introduction

Chronic pain is a significant public health problem. Chronic pain conditions are highly prevalent, costly and can be disabling. Over 100 million Americans are estimated to experience chronic pain at any given time.[179] Conservative estimates place measurable loss in productivity and direct costs due to chronic pain at over $500 billion annually.[179] Chronic pain conditions are a leading cause of disability globally.[150] US adults frequently seek care outside of mainstream medical practices to treat pain. The term "complementary health approaches" refers broadly to therapeutic practices that have their origins outside of conventional Western and allopathic medical traditions;[203] these include practices such as yoga, herbal supplements and hypnosis. Some complementary approaches are quite mainstream today and commonly used by Americans.[204]

There is no widely agreed upon self-report instrument for use of complementary health approaches and other common conventional non-pharmacological techniques for pain and health management. Past efforts to standardize reported usage of complementary health approaches have not been widely adopted.[205] Lack of standardization complicates comparing results between studies[186] because any estimate of complementary health approach utilization in a population will depend on what is included in an investigator's list of modalities. Additionally, there are no widely-endorsed classification schemes for individual complementary health approaches. The National Center for

Complementary and Integrative Health (NCCIH) has broadly classified practices as Mind and Body, Natural Products, and Others.[206] The National Center for Health Statistics (NCHS) has classified approaches as Natural Products, Practitioner-based, Mind and Body, or Whole Medical Systems.[156] Even the categories that share the same name do not contain the same list of practices. For example, in the NCCIH taxonomy, chiropractic, acupuncture, and yoga are all "Mind and Body;" whereas in the NCHS taxonomy, chiropractic is "Practitioner-based," acupuncture is "Whole Medical Systems," and yoga is "Mind and Body."

Nearly one-third of US adults have used any complementary health approach in the previous 12 months.[186] Much of what is known broadly about people who use complementary health approaches in the US comes from the 2002, 2007 and 2012 National Health Interview Survey (NHIS), so its classification scheme is especially relevant.[207] Since the first iteration in 2002, complementary modalities that were mostly understood to be delivered by a practitioner were preceded by the question stem, "Have you ever seen a practitioner for..."; whereas self-directed modalities had the stem, "Have you ever used...".[207(p11)] This categorization was developed following initial cognitive interviewing that found survey respondents generally experienced complementary practices differently if they did them independently versus seeing a practitioner for them.[207(p11)] This broad taxonomy has been subdivided by various authors but nonetheless persists in the way questions are asked of NHIS respondents. Elsewhere, self-directed complementary approaches have been referred to as active and that terminology here is adopted here.[65]

This study was developed to address several gaps in the literature. First, there is a need for a standardized self-report inventory of common non-pharmacological therapies to facilitate interpretability of results between studies. Second, it is unclear if existing categorization schemes would emerge from an analysis of actual patterns of use in a sample of complementary users. Third, it has not been documented how practitioner-delivered and active complementary practices may overlap with practitioner-delivered and active conventional practices. Evidence suggests people are not using complementary health approaches in isolation but rather with other complementary and conventional modalities.[208] Though the demographics of complementary therapy users have been well-characterized in different contexts, less is known about the contribution of psychological traits in adoption of complementary practices.[133] Anxiety, depression and worse self-rated psychological health may be more prevalent in people who use complementary approaches than those who do not.[209] Little is known about absorption (the capacity for dedicating one's full attention to the senses and imagination and becoming deeply immersed in those attentional experiences), one of 11 personality scales measured by the Multidimensional Personality Questionnaire.[104,130] Absorption is related to openness to experience, but is distinct. Openness to experience has been shown to be positively associated with use of and belief in complementary therapies.[132,133]

To address these gaps, a checklist was created that included conventional and complementary non-pharmacological approaches employed in multimodal pain management—the Health Practices Inventory—and it was tested in a sample of National Guard veterans of Operation Iraqi Freedom (OIF), Operation Enduring Freedom (OEF), and Operation New Dawn (OND). The aims of this study were: 1) develop and pilot the Health Practices Inventory; 2) identify groupings of complementary and conventional pain management approaches by latent class analysis and compare to the *a priori* categorization of active versus practitioner-delivered; 3) estimate associations between sociodemographic, psychological, behavioral and pain covariates and the predicted latent classes of complementary use patterns.

L.2. Methods

L.2.i. *Development of Health Practices Inventory*

The Health Practices Inventory (HPI) is a self-report checklist designed to assess use of non-pharmacological approaches for pain management or other reasons (Figure L-2, p. 119). The HPI covers 19 well-described active and practitioner-delivered complementary and conventional modalities, based on the classification proposed by NCCIH[156,207] and the Active Self-Care Therapies for Pain Working Group[65] (see Table L-1, p. 112, for classifications). The 19 modalities were purposefully selected to represent non-pharmacological approaches that are commonly used for chronic pain. An initial list of 28 modalities was developed from examination of the contents of the NHIS complementary and alternative medicine (CAM) supplement and review of specific modalities included in other questionnaires, by examining frequently available complementary therapies in the VA healthcare system,[210] and by surveying the pain literature, including guidelines for pain management approaches. Definitions of each modality were prepared by reviewing interview questions from the NHIS CAM supplement[211] and the publicly available sections of the NCCIH website.[204] Two clinician authors (MAP and EEK) consulted with Dr. Barbara Stussman from the NCCIH, who provided feedback on the initial draft. EEK conducted key informant interviews with four experts in complementary and conventional pain management to shorten the initial list of 28 modalities and refine their definitions.

Respondents were asked to indicate whether they had used each modality in the past year for health reasons. For each modality endorsed, respondents were asked to indicate their reason(s) for use (improve well-being/general health, manage pain, or manage a condition other than pain, not mutually exclusive) and to rate the frequency of use in the past month (not at all, several days, more than half the days, nearly every day). A summary variable for each of 4 main categories of HPI modalities (i.e. active complementary, active conventional, practitioner-delivered complementary, other complementary) and use of these categories was dichotomized as yes/no for using any modality in that category. Overall use of complementary modalities was assessed as the number of different active and practitioner-delivered complementary modalities reported by each respondent.

L.2.ii. *Cognitive Interviewing.* One study investigator conducted cognitive interviews using a preliminary version of the HPI with five veterans. Participants were sent a questionnaire by mail and instructed to complete it in one sitting, marking any items that were confusing or raised questions. A semi-structured cognitive interview was then conducted. Interviews used a flexible set of probing questions and targeted follow-up questions that enabled the interviewer to gather more in-depth information based on participants' responses.

Following recommendations for cognitive interviewing outlined by Willis,[212,213] probing questions focused on assessing: 1) the participant's comprehension of the questions, 2) the participant's ability to adequately recall the information needed to respond to the questions, 3) the level of cognitive processing required to answer the questions, and 4) the participant's ability to match his/her internally generated answer with the response options given on the survey. To assess whether participants answered questions as intended by investigators, they were instructed to "think aloud" and describe the process they went through to answer certain questions. The cognitive interviewing process largely confirmed comprehension and clarity of HPI items. Only minor changes were made after the cognitive interviewing process.

L.2.iii. *Procedures and Participants*

Data are from a single wave of follow-up data from the Readiness and Resilience in National Guard Soldiers (RINGS)[139] Study, a longitudinal cohort study originally designed to identify predictors of post-deployment health experiences of OIF/OEF/OND veterans. The eligible RINGS cohort included

3,890 Army National Guard Soldiers deployed to OIF, OEF, or OND between 2006 and 2011 who were assessed prior to or during deployment and completed at least one post-deployment assessment. The data for this manuscript come from the most recent follow-up survey administered from October 2015 to September 2016.

Respondents were administered a battery of self-report measures assessing pain, comorbid mental health symptoms (including PTSD, depression, anxiety, and substance abuse), overall health-related quality of life, and health services utilization. Data were collected using standard mailed survey methodology.[172] A follow-up questionnaire, cover letter containing all elements of informed consent, and $20 incentive were mailed to 3,843 panel members (42 had untrackable addresses, 1 was incarcerated, and 4 were deceased). A postcard reminder and two additional survey mailings were sent to non-responders at 2 week intervals, with the final mailing delivered by priority mail. The overall response rate was 48.1% (n=1,850). Demographics of all eligible cohort members were recorded from administrative records. Non-responders were very similar to the responders. The non-responders were slightly younger than responders and less likely to be female. All study procedures were approved by the institutional review boards of the Minneapolis VA Medical Center and University of Minnesota. A waiver of documentation of informed consent was approved for this study by both IRBs.

Veterans listed in the RINGS registry were informed about RINGS-CAM through a study newsletter, which provides updates on the ongoing longitudinal study. After 2 to 3 weeks, an initial survey packet was sent to all eligible Veterans. The packet included an informed consent letter detailing the study, their rights to withdraw or refuse, and venues for asking any questions. Veterans could refuse to take part in this study at any time by calling a toll-free number included in the pre-notification letter or returning their survey blank. At 2-week intervals, eligible participants who had not yet responded were mailed a reminder postcard, a second mailed questionnaire, and a final third questionnaire sent by priority mail.

L.2.iv.   *Measures*

Pain. Chronic pain was defined as experiencing pain on at least half the days of the previous 6 months. This definition follows from the recommendations from the National Pain Strategy.[194] Characteristic pain intensity and interference was measured by the 3-item PEG scale.[193]

Mental Health. Anxiety symptoms were measured using the 8-item PROMIS short form 8a anxiety scale[174] (Patient Reported Outcomes Measurement Information System). The scale was dichotomized at 22 (corresponding to a T-score >60),[214] above which scores are consistent with moderate or severe anxiety. Depressive symptoms were measured with the 8-item Patient Health Questionnaire depression scale (PHQ-8).[87] The PHQ-8 was dichotomized at 10,[87] consistent with a positive screen for depression. Post-traumatic stress symptoms were measured with the PTSD Checklist-5 (PCL-5).[118] The PCL-5 was dichotomized at 33, consistent with probable PTSD.[118] The personality dimension of absorption was measured using the Brief Form of the Multidimensional Personality Questionnaire 12-item absorption subscale.[104,130]

Substance use. Illicit drug use was measured with the Drug Abuse Screening Test (DAST).[90] A score above 0 represents any illicit drug use in the previous year. Alcohol use was measured with the Alcohol Use Disorders Identification Test (AUDIT).[128] The AUDIT score was dichotomized above 7, consistent with problem alcohol use.[128]

Self-rated health. Overall health was self-reported using the single-item global heath and 1-year prior health questions from the Veterans RAND 12 Item Health Survey (VR-12).[195,196] Overall health was dichotomized as excellent/very good versus good/fair/poor. "Physical health worse" is a self-report of slightly worse or much worse (vs much better/slightly better/about the same) physical health compared to one year ago. "Emotional problems worse" is a self-report of slightly worse or much worse (vs much better/slightly better/about the same) emotional problems compared to one year ago.

Demographics. Age was recorded at time of survey mailing from an administrative record. Participants were asked in this survey to report gender, race, ethnicity, educational attainment, employment, deployment experiences and length of military service. To assess past combat exposure, participants were asked, "During any deployment, were you ever a participant or observer in direct combat operations?" They could respond, "Yes, participated in direct combat operation(s)", or "Yes, observed or witnessed combat operation(s)," or "No." These three options were analyzed as mutually exclusive. To assess deployment injuries, participants were asked to recall, "Were you wounded or injured during any deployment?" They could respond, "Yes" or "No."

L.2.v.   *Statistical Analyses*

Latent class analysis was used to identify distinct subgroups of use of conventional and complementary non-pharmacological therapies for health management. Latent class analysis is an exploratory data reduction technique that categorizes respondents into multiple discrete, non-overlapping classes based on similar patterns of observed data. Because the classes are latent, they cannot be directly observed and can only be estimated using observed response patterns. The purpose of the latent class analysis in this study was to combine the responses to the 19 HPI approaches into a small number of substantively meaningful classes about which inferences could be made. For a latent class analysis with binary data, as in this study, the model estimates the probability that a member of each class endorses each item. Estimates from the latent class model were used to calculate the probability an individual was in a class as a function of their actual response pattern.

Frequency of modality use was dichotomized as any use versus no use in the previous 12 months. Fewer than 2% of respondents reported using biofeedback, Tai Chi/Qi Gong, Healing Touch/Reiki, homeopathy, and hypnotherapy; including these rare approaches led to estimability problems, so they were excluded from the latent class analysis. The latent class model used only self-report of individual HPI modalities to predict class membership. Separate models were fit with 1 to 11 latent classes. The fit of these models was compared using the Bayesian Information Criterion and Akaike's Information Criterion. The best-fitting latent class model had 6 distinct and substantively meaningful classes (see Table L-2, p. 114, for model fit statistics). Respondents each had a posterior probability of class membership calculated and were assigned class membership according to their maximum class probability. Sociodemographic, psychological distress, and substance use items, as well as absorption and the dichotomous 6-month chronic pain item, were then used as predictors in a multinomial regression model with the latent classes as outcomes. Marginal effects (i.e. difference in class membership probabilities) were calculated from the regression results by standardizing the distribution of covariates to their distribution in the total sample and calculating the difference in probability of class membership between levels of the covariate.[215] All analyses were performed in Stata 15.[176]

L.2.vi.   *Missing Data*

Approximately 14% of respondents had missing data for at least one predictor. To address the concern that this missingness could bias results, 20 datasets were imputed by chained multiple imputation to allow all respondents to be included.[216–218] Continuous measures and ordered scales were imputed by predictive mean matching with 5 nearest neighbors and imputed values were drawn from 20 independent bootstrap samples.[219,220] Continuous measures were dichotomized after imputation. Binary and factor variables were imputed by logistic regression or multinomial logistic regression. All imputed variables were included in the chained equations and maximum probability latent class was included as a fixed (not imputed) variable. The scales that were not included in the multinomial logistic regression were still included in the chained imputation equations to improve performance of the imputation.

L.3. Results

Table L-3 (p. 115) presents demographic characteristics of respondents as well as mean scores on self-report scales. Respondents were mostly male, white and 36 years old or younger. According to study definitions, 41% had chronic pain and 22% had a positive depression screen.

Table L-1 (p. 112) summarizes the responses to the HPI by all respondents. Data on past-year use of all 19 HPI modalities were complete for 1,816 respondents (98%); the HPI past-year use items were completely skipped by 25 respondents (1%); 6 respondents skipped past-year use for 1 of the modalities (<1%); 2 respondents skipped several of the past-year items (<1%). Seventy-four percent endorsed use of at least one HPI modality in the 12 months prior to the survey; 57% endorsed any active conventional approach, 26% endorsed any active complementary approach, and 44% endorsed any practitioner-delivered complementary approach. The most commonly reported complementary approaches were chiropractic care (31.7% of all respondents) and massage (23.6%). Respondents in this study most commonly reported engaging with active conventional approaches and endorsed well-being/general health as the main reason for using them.

Of those endorsing use of any practitioner-delivered complementary approach, 76.2% reported using it for pain, compared with 24.2% of those using any active complementary approach, 18.6% using any other complementary approach, and 28.4% using active conventional approaches. Active complementary (72.6%), other complementary (79.9%), and active conventional approaches (79.5%) were more commonly reported for well-being/general health (versus 42.3% for practitioner-delivered complementary). Active conventional (42.8%) and other complementary (60.1%) approaches were most likely to be used daily. Active complementary was most commonly used several days a month (52.2%) and practitioner-delivered complementary was most likely to be used less than monthly (48.1%).

Table L-4 (p. 116) presents the prevalence of use of the HPI modalities within the 6 classes. The 6 classes were named to reflect the distinguishing prevalence of modalities between classes. One class represented very low rates of HPI use, "Low users" (50% of respondents, n=923). Five classes represented higher rates of HPI use (the 5 HPI-use classes): "Exercise users" (23%, n=426), "Psychotherapy users" (5%, n=87), "Chiropractic & massage users" (12%, n=213), "Mindfulness & relaxation users" (7%, n=126), and "High users multimodal" (4%, n=75). The 6 classes identified in the best-fit latent class model were robust across other latent class model solutions with different numbers of classes. Notably, the Low users, Exercise users and Psychotherapy users classes were easy to identify in the next best-fit models (5 and 7 classes). The major differences were in how the complementary classes were divided. With 7 classes, the Chiropractic & massage users class was split into two classes, one with high rates of strengthening/stretching and aerobic exercise and one with low rates of exercise. With 5 classes, the Mindfulness & relaxation users class and High users multimodal class merged into one class.

All class members in the Chiropractic & massage users, Mindfulness & relaxation users, and High users multimodal classes reported use of any complementary modality, compared with 31% of members of the low modality users class. Nearly three-quarters of the sample had at least some engagement with HPI modalities, yet half were best classified as low modality users. The remaining respondents reported mixed use of conventional and complementary approaches, with an average of 2 different complementary approaches over the past year. The High users multimodal class had the highest median overall use of complementary approaches (median=5; SE: 0.1). The Chiropractic & massage users (median=2; SE: 0.06), Mindfulness & relaxation users (median=2; SE: 0.1) and Psychotherapy users classes (median=2; SE: 0.1) had similar medians but less than the highest. The Exercise users class (median=1; SE: 0.04) and Low users class (median=0; SE: 0.02) had the least.

The practitioner-delivered complementary and active complementary modalities tended to cluster within their *a priori* categories. The Chiropractic & massage users class used practitioner-delivered complementary modalities at a higher proportion than the total sample and active complementary modalities at rates similar to those of the total sample. Similarly, the Mindfulness & relaxation class used active complementary modalities at a higher rate than the total sample (with the exception of yoga) and practitioner-delivered complementary at rates similar to the total sample. The "Other complementary" approaches were highly used only by the High users multimodal class.

Figure L-1 (p. 118) presents estimates of the effect of each covariate on probability of membership in each of the latent classes, compared to low modality users. A positive value means that being in the named level of the covariate of that row increases the probability of membership in that latent class instead of the Low users class. For example, having obtained a 4-year degree instead of no 4-year degree is associated with a 0.14 increased prevalence of the Exercise users class relative to the Low modality users class. Also, a positive screen for problem alcohol use instead of a negative screen is associated with a 0.08 decrease in the prevalence of the Chiropractic & massage users class compared to the Low users class. Higher education is positively associated with membership in the Exercise users class and problem alcohol use is negatively associated with membership in the Chiropractic & massage users class, compared to the Low users class.

Higher absorption and higher education were generally associated with higher prevalence of the five HPI-use classes (compared to the Low users class); only the Psychotherapy users class was not associated with higher education and only the Chiropractic & massage users class was not associated with higher absorption. Depression was not associated with any of the 5 HPI-use classes. PTSD was only associated with the Psychotherapy class and problem alcohol use was only (negatively) associated with the Chiropractic & massage users class. This means that some of the covariates better distinguish between classes and some of the covariates better predict higher rates of HPI use broadly.

Each class had a unique set of covariates that were associated with a difference in prevalence compared to the Low modality users class. For example, higher anxiety was associated with the Psychotherapy users class and the High users multimodal class, but higher anxiety with higher PTSD distinguishes the Psychotherapy users class from the High users multimodal class. Chronic pain was associated with the Chiropractic & massage users class and the High users multimodal class. But chronic pain with higher absorption distinguishes the High users multimodal class from the Chiropractic & massage users class. Both the Chiropractic & massage users class and the Mindfulness & relaxation users class are associated with higher education and higher illicit drug use, but the Chiropractic & massage users class is distinguished by being female and having chronic pain and the Mindfulness & relaxation users class is distinguished by higher absorption and better self-rated health.

L.4. Discussion

Our study has shown that complementary and conventional non-pharmacological therapies are being used together and in distinct patterns with unique sets of predictors. Most people who use complementary approaches are also using conventional approaches at similar rates to the general population. Active conventional approaches are being used without complementary approaches by nearly a quarter of the sample, but the particular conventional approaches being used differ between classes of HPI users. The way complementary and conventional approaches are being integrated identify unique classes of users of non-pharmacological health approaches. An exception was chiropractic, some of the users of which were not also using conventional approaches.

In the current study, the most commonly reported modality used for pain was chiropractic care. This is consistent with estimates in the civilian US adult population—which show that practitioner-delivered complementary are used more frequently than active complementary practices—and with Midwestern regional trends in higher use of chiropractic.[221] This is also consistent with the availability of services for military and veterans.[222] Herman et al. reported that military medical facilities that offered complementary approaches were most likely to offer chiropractic, acupuncture or multimodal complementary approaches for pain, but active complementary approaches were more likely to be offered than practitioner-delivered complementary approaches for conditions other than pain including anxiety, stress and PTSD. In a broader sense, clinical guidelines and the evidence base do not provide support for favoring practitioner-delivered complementary approaches for pain management over active ones, except possibly in acute pain.[13,159,223]

Prior studies have found that use of complementary health approaches is greater among women, middle age groups, people with more education and higher income, and people reporting a musculoskeletal pain disorder.[156,186] Yet presenting the characteristics of users of any complementary approaches, in aggregate, may mask important trends within categories.[224] These analyses illustrate distinct patterns in the use of conventional and complementary health approaches among respondents. Though most of the sample would be characterized as complementary users by a simple binary indicator, these results show heterogeneity in type of complementary therapy use and that demographic, psychological and behavioral predictors of use vary between the distinct patterns of use. For example, use of active complementary modalities was best predicted by higher anxiety whereas use of practitioner-delivered complementary modalities was predicted by chronic pain. Higher use of non-pharmacological therapies generally was predicted by female sex, higher educational attainment, and higher absorption.

Our results support the previously developed categorizations of active versus practitioner-delivered complementary modalities; these categories also emerged statistically in the latent class analysis. The observation in 2002 that people experience active and practitioner-delivered complementary approaches differently can be again observed from these findings. The difference between active and practitioner-delivered modalities appears to be functionally important as there is a clear distinction in why people use these types of modalities. Participants in this survey were far more likely to report using practitioner-delivered complementary approaches for pain rather than well-being, and far more likely to report using active complementary approaches for well-being rather than pain. Additionally, participants are using active complementary approaches far more often than practitioner-delivered approaches; however, fewer participants overall are using active complementary approaches compared to practitioner-delivered complementary approaches.

There is a noticeable gap in the literature when it comes to absorption, one of 11 personality scales measured by the Multidimensional Personality Questionnaire. It can be briefly described as the capacity for dedicating one's full attention to the senses and imagination and becoming deeply immersed in those attentional experiences.[130] It is historically tied to complementary medicine because it was originally designed as a predictive measure of response to hypnosis (a complementary modality). Since absorption is positively correlated with openness to experience yet distinct, it is an intriguing personality dimension to study. Openness to experience has been shown to be positively associated with use of and belief in complementary therapies.[132,133] A recent systematic review[132] of traits and cognitions as predictors of complementary approach use and beliefs identified only two small published studies that reported on absorption. Both studies found unadjusted moderate positive correlations between absorption and using complementary approaches. Those findings are consistent with those of the present study. Moreover, these results add to the understanding of absorption as an independent predictor of complementary approach use with a more sophisticated analysis controlling for sociodemographic variables, pain, distress and externalizing behaviors.

This study has several limitations. First, although the HPI allows collection of detailed data about how often and why respondents use non-pharmacological therapies, modality use was dichotomized as any versus no use in the past year, which statistically equates daily use and one-time use. Practice use was dichotomized because when frequency was included, the groups seemed to be defined by frequency of exercise, not patterns of use of the other modalities, which did not suit the purposes of this study. A second limitation is survey non-response. If nonresponders are substantially different from responders, the results may have been different had nonresponders been included; however, study administrative records show that the nonresponders are quite similar to those who responded, which could mitigate this problem. Another source of missing data was item missingness. Multiple imputation to address this in the multinomial logistic regression and results were consistent with complete case analysis. An additional limitation is the possibility of misclassification. If respondents to the HPI did not correctly identify the practices they used, they may be classified inappropriately and added to the wrong latent class. Also, the associations between the predictor covariates and latent class membership from the multinomial logistic regression may be biased by unmeasured confounding. These limitations combined could create associations where there were none in actuality or mask associations that truly are there. Finally, the demographic characteristics of US adults who use complementary health approaches do not align well with those of most veterans receiving VA health care.[225] At the same time, US veterans report higher use of complementary approaches than do US civilians.[226,227] It is possible that the predictors of use are different in this sample that US adults in general, therefore it is important that these findings be replicated in other civilian samples.

The HPI is an efficient way to collect useful data on use of non-pharmacological therapies for well-being and managing pain and other medical conditions. The practical categories of practitioner-delivered versus active in both complementary and conventional approaches are emergent in the patterns of use in a sample of recently deployed veterans. Additionally, people combining practitioner-delivered and active complementary approaches represent a distinct population of complementary users. This is significant because many analyses do not acknowledge both distinct and combined-use groups. These findings should be investigated in other contexts and with other samples. In particular, additional latent class analyses with new samples could provide evidence for or against these 6 classes. Additionally, further studies are justified to explore the role of absorption in uptake of complementary practices.

This paper is a novel application of latent class analysis to demonstrate heterogeneity in how people are using complementary and conventional approaches together for their health. This analysis has shown the value of treating these heterogeneous classes of use separately to discover important differences in the variables that are associated with the different classes. Collapsing these groups of complementary modality users would hide clinical meaningful differences in overall health, chronic pain, and psychological distress. Investigators should use caution when collapsing active and practitioner-delivered complementary modalities into one "complementary and integrative health" class. Other teams are encouraged to use the Health Practices Inventory to report usage of non-pharmacological approaches for health management in their studies.

L.5. Tables and Figures

Table L-1: Self-reported past-year use of Health Practices Inventory approaches (N=1,825)

Type of modality	%	(n)	Reason for use† Well-being/ general health %	Treat pain %	Treat another condition %	Past month Frequency of use‡ None %	Several days %	More %
Active complementary modalities								
Relaxation	18.4	(335)	63.3	19.4	37.3	12.5	54.3	25.1
Mindfulness/Meditation	10.4	(190)	73.7	11.6	31.6	10.0	52.1	24.7
Yoga	9.5	(174)	85.1	33.3	13.8	31.0	50.0	8.1
Biofeedback	1.6	(30)	70.0	13.3	16.7	46.7	33.3	13.3
Tai Chi/Qi Gong	0.8	(15)	86.7	33.3	6.7	26.7	33.3	13.3
Any active complementary*	26.0	(475)	72.6	24.2	31.6	15.4	52.2	23.0
Practitioner-delivered complementary								
Chiropractic	31.7	(578)	31	82.5	8.1	46.4	46.0	2.4
Massage	23.6	(431)	52.4	63.1	8.1	56.2	33.4	2.1
Acupuncture	4.7	(86)	37.2	72.1	22.1	68.6	27.9	0.0
Reiki/Healing Touch	1.2	(21)	52.4	52.4	38.1	47.6	42.9	4.8
Any practitioner-delivered complementary	43.7	(797)	42.3	76.2	10.7	48.1	43.9	2.9
Other complementary modalities								
Herbal supplement	9.6	(175)	80	15.4	19.4	4.6	26.3	60
Diet	6.6	(120)	76.7	20.8	19.2	9.2	17.5	63.3
Spiritual/traditional healing system	6.3	(115)	78.3	13.9	28.7	9.6	39.1	44.4
Homeopathy	1.4	(25)	60	44	40	36	32	28
Hypnotherapy	0.5	(9)	33.3	22.2	44.4	66.7	0	22.2
Any Other complementary	18.3	(338)	79.9	18.6	24.9	8.4	24.0	60.1
Active conventional modalities								
Strength/stretch exercise	43.8	(799)	75.6	33.7	9.8	8.6	37.1	45.1
Aerobic exercise	36.2	(661)	87.8	12.1	8.5	4.2	42.1	45.4
Psychotherapy	12.8	(233)	53.7	9.4	49.8	39.1	45.9	5.2
Any active conventional	57.0	(1040)	79.5	28.4	18.4	10.2	39.4	42.8
Practitioner-delivered conventional modalities								
Manual physical therapy	13.3	(242)	15.3	79.8	12.4	41.3	43.4	8.3
Other conventional modalities								
Support groups	4.3	(79)	62.0	7.6	39.2	30.4	45.6	12.7

Table L-1: Self-reported past-year use of Health Practices Inventory approaches (N=1,825)

*The Health Practices Inventory approaches are grouped based on the *a priori* categorization described in the text; a summary variable was created for each of the groupings indicating use of any of the modalities in that group

†Respondents who reported using a Health Practices Inventory modality were asked to identify their reason(s) for using it; the reasons are not mutually exclusive and they could pick any combination of the three reasons listed or none at all

‡Respondents who reported using a Health Practices Inventory modality were asked to identify the frequency they used it in the past month; these frequencies are mutually exclusive but do not always add up to 100% because of missingness

Table L-2: Comparison of the different model fit statistics examined to determine the best fitting model (best number of classes). BIC was the primary statistic used, with % success as a key measure of achieving the correct model solution.

No. classes	LL	AIC	aBIC	BIC	CAIC	S	% success
1	-10165	20357	20390	20435	20449	1.000	100%
2	-9416	18890	18957	19049	19078	0.707	100%
3	-9206	18498	18598	18735	18778	0.597	98%
4	-9111	18337	18472	18657	18715	0.517	39%
5	-9020	18186	18356	18588	18661	0.429	91%
6	-8971	18110	18306	18573	18657	0.455	42%
7	-8943	18071	18288	18583	18676	0.387	31%
8	-8918	18039	18277	18601	18703	0.372	1%
9	-8893	18020	18293	18665	18782	0.313	1%
10	-8873	18002	18300	18707	18835	0.222	2%
11	-8851	17971	18283	18709	18843	0.164	1%

Table L-3: Characteristics of respondents to the mailed survey

Characteristic	Respondents
Male, % (N)	90.3% (1668)
Age, Mean (SD)	38.7 (9.2)
White, % (N)	90.1% (1656)
Obtained 4-year degree, % (N)	42.6% (772)
Injured on deployment, % (N)	27.0% (493)
Pain	
Chronic pain, % (N)	41.2% (749)
Intensity and interference (PEG), Mean (SD)	2.4 (2.4)
Self-rated health, % (N)	
Current health excellent/very good*	43.1% (796)
Physical health worse†	28.1% (513)
Emotional problems worse†	25.7% (468)
Mental health, % (N)	
Anxiety at least moderate (PROMIS-Anxiety 8a ≥ 22)	21.8% (400)
Depression (PHQ-8 ≥ 10)	21.7% (392)
Probable PTSD (PCL-5 ≥ 33)	19.5% (339)
Substance use, % (N)	
Problem alcohol use (AUDIT ≥ 8)	21.6% (394)
Past year illicit drug use (DAST > 0)	10.3% (184)
Absorption (MPQ-BF Absorption, T-scores), Mean (SD)	47.6 (10.8)

Abbreviations PEG: 3-item PEG scale; VR-12: Veterans RAND 12-Item Health Survey

* Current health excellent/very good vs good/fair/poor; VR-12 overall health item

† Self-reported physical health worse/emotional problems worse, compared to last year. Items 8 and 9, respectively, from the VR-12

Table L-4: Probability of use of Health Practices Inventory approaches within latent classes of respondents to mailed survey (N = 1,850)

	Low use (50%, n=923)	Exercise (23%, n=426)	Psychotherapy (6%, n=112)	Chiropractic & massage (12%, n=213)	Mindfulness & relaxation (5%, n=101)	High use multimodal (4%, n=75)	Total use** (100%, n=1850)
Relaxation*	4%#	13%	65%	13%	83%	89%	18%
Mindfulness/ Meditation*	1%	0%	42%	4%	100%	52%	10%
Yoga*	1%	12%	4%	15%	34%	47%	9.5%
Chiropractic†	22%	23%	26%	78%	10%	70%	32%
Massage†	7%	22%	32%	64%	28%	76%	24%
Acupuncture†	1%	0%	11%	21%	0%	20%	4.7%
Herbal supplements‡	1%	14%	1%	17%	22%	49%	9.6%
Diet‡	0%	12%	2%	8%	12%	41%	6.6%
Spiritual Healing‡	1%	9%	18%	4%	13%	39%	6.3%
Strength/stretch exercise§	11%	86%	28%	61%	74%	97%	44%
Aerobic exercise§	5%	86%	18%	40%	69%	78%	36%
Psychotherapy§	6%	9%	79%	11%	14%	28%	13%
Manual physical therapy‖	6%	9%	25%	35%	4%	49%	13%
Support groups¶	1%	2%	49%	0%	2%	12%	4.3%

Lower use ··· Higher Use

Table L-4: Probability of use of Health Practices Inventory approaches within latent classes of respondents to mailed survey (N = 1,850)

*Classified as active complementary modality by expert classification

†Classified as practitioner-delivered complementary modality

‡Classified as Other complementary modality

§Classified as active conventional modality

‖Classified as practitioner-delivered conventional modality

¶Classified as Other conventional modality

**Bolding** added to highlight proportions that distinguish classes; all proportions that represent an odds ratio greater than 5 or less than 0.2 compared to use among all responders were considered much higher or much lower use than in the total sample and were **bolded and underlined**

** Total use represents the proportion of use of modalities in the total sample. This is not a latent class.

Figure L-1: Table of effects of covariates on prevalence of latent classes compared to low use class; results of multinomial regression

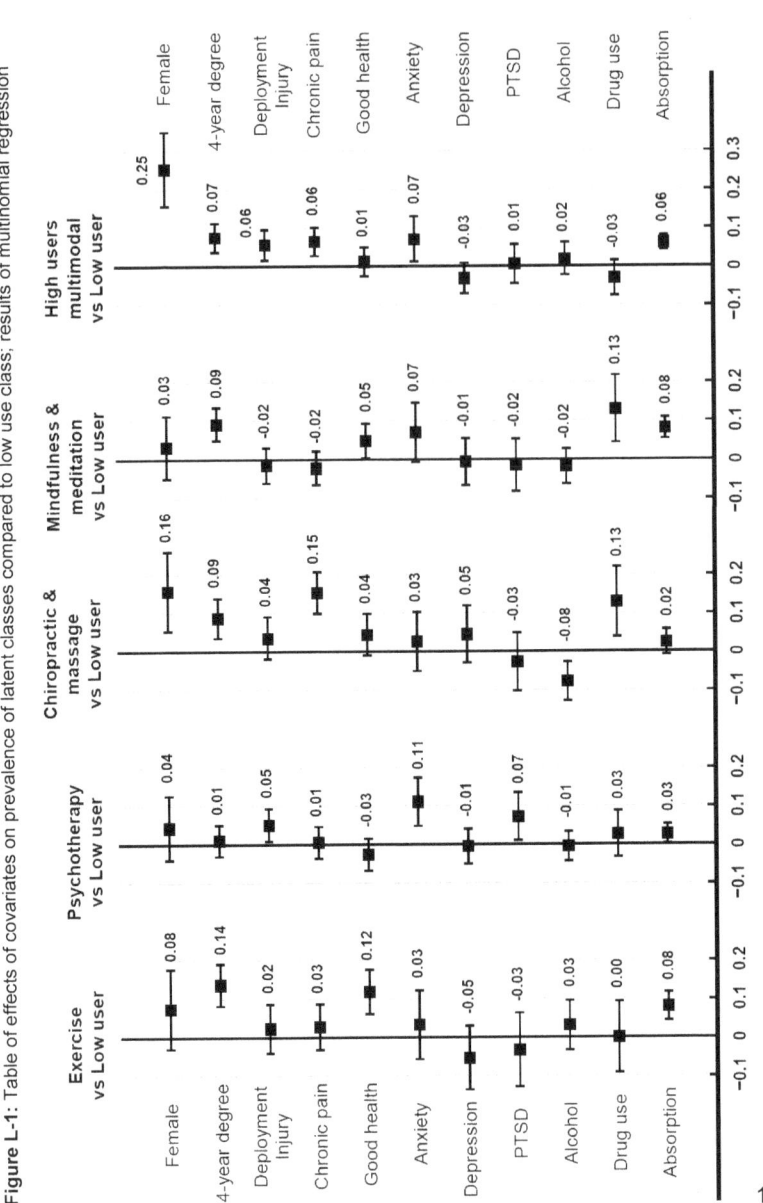

118

Figure L-2: Full text of the Health Practices Inventory

SECTION E: TELL US ABOUT YOUR HEALTH CARE EXPERIENCES

Below is a list of treatments, practices, and services that people use for health reasons. Please tell us if you have used each one in the past year by marking "Yes" or "No." If you mark "Yes," please tell us why and how often you have used the treatment.

In the past year, I have used...		If yes, why? *Choose all that apply.*			How often in the past month?			
		Improve well-being/ general health	Manage pain	Manage a condition other than pain	Not at all	Several days	More than half the days	Nearly every day
Acupuncture: Stimulation of specific points of the body, with thin needles.	○ Yes → ○ No	○	○	○	○	○	○	○
Biofeedback: Use of sensors to teach control over body functions such as breathing, heart rate and muscle tone.	○ Yes → ○ No	○	○	○	○	○	○	○
Chiropractic: Hands on adjustment of spine and joints to improve alignment, function, or pain.	○ Yes → ○ No	○	○	○	○	○	○	○
Massage Therapy: Hands on pressure, rubbing, or manipulation of muscles and soft tissues.	○ Yes → ○ No	○	○	○	○	○	○	○
Rehabilitation Therapies: Hands on treatment such as traction, TENS, ultrasound, or mobilization by a PT or OT to treat pain or injury.	○ Yes → ○ No	○	○	○	○	○	○	○
Healing/Therapeutic Touch or Reiki: Gentle techniques to alter energy fields and restore balance to allow healing.	○ Yes → ○ No	○	○	○	○	○	○	○
Hypnosis/Hypnotherapy: Use of deep relaxation and power of suggestion to change responses and behaviors.	○ Yes → ○ No	○	○	○	○	○	○	○
Psychotherapy: One-on-one or group talk therapy, such as cognitive behavioral therapy (CBT), by a psychologist or other mental health provider.	○ Yes → ○ No	○	○	○	○	○	○	○
Support Group: A therapeutic group formed around a shared problem or experience.	○ Yes → ○ No	○	○	○	○	○	○	○
Spiritual or Traditional Healing: Use of faith-based, religious, or spiritual practice to promote health or healing.	○ Yes → ○ No	○	○	○	○	○	○	○

Figure L-2: Full text of the Health Practices Inventory *(continued)*

SECTION E: TELL US ABOUT YOUR HEALTH CARE EXPERIENCES

Below is a list of treatments, practices, and services that people use for health reasons. Please tell us if you have used each one in the past year by marking "Yes" or "No." If you mark "Yes," please tell us why and how often you have used the treatment.

In *the past year*, I have used...		If yes, why? *Choose all that apply.*			How often in the past month?			
		Improve well-being/ general health	Manage pain	Manage a condition other than pain	Not at all	Several days	More than half the days	Nearly every day
Relaxation Techniques: Use of breathing, guided imagery, or progressive muscle relaxation to cause a relaxation response.	○ Yes → ○ No	○	○	○	○	○	○	○
Meditation/Mindfulness Practice: Use of focused attention and non-judgmental awareness, including transcendental, mindfulness meditation, Mindfulness Based Stress Reduction.	○ Yes → ○ No	○	○	○	○	○	○	○
Yoga: Practices that combine physical postures, breathing techniques, and meditation or relaxation.	○ Yes → ○ No	○	○	○	○	○	○	○
Tai Chi/Qi Gong: Combined practice of slow movements, coordinated-breathing, and mental focus.	○ Yes → ○ No	○	○	○	○	○	○	○
Stretching/Strengthening Exercise Therapy: Training or home exercise program using stretches or weights to improve flexibility, posture, or strength.	○ Yes → ○ No	○	○	○	○	○	○	○
Aerobic Exercise Therapy: Training or home exercise program using activities such as walking, swimming or aerobics to increase fitness or edurance.	○ Yes → ○ No	○	○	○	○	○	○	○
Diet-based Therapies: Use of specific diet for health purposes, such as anti-inflammatory.	○ Yes → ○ No	○	○	○	○	○	○	○
Herbal Supplements: Use of plant-based, herb, or botanical product such as echinacea.	○ Yes → ○ No	○	○	○	○	○	○	○
Homeopathy: Individualized treatment by a homeopathic practioner or use of homeopathic remedies.	○ Yes → ○ No	○	○	○	○	○	○	○

Table L-5: Comparison of characteristics of survey respondents and non-respondents

Characteristic	Responders (n = 1,850)	Non-responders (n = 1,993)
Male, % (N)	90.5 (1,638)	92.1 (1,744)
Age, Mean (SD)	38.7 (9.2)	33.5 (7.9)
White, % (N)	93.8 (1,592)	92.9 (1,658)
Lives in urban area, % (N)	51.6 (933)	52.0 (985)
Eligible for VA healthcare, % (N)	59.2 (1,071)	51.9 (982)
Anxiety-related diagnosis from VA within past year, % (N)	9.4 (174)	11.4 (225)
Depression-related diagnosis from VA within past year, % (N)	11.2 (208)	11.9 (235)
PTSD diagnosis from VA within past year, % (N)	13.0 (242)	11.7 (231)

Abbreviations: VA: Veterans Affairs

Table L-6: Prevalence differences of class membership due to covariates; results of multinomial logistic regression

Covariate*	Exercise users vs. Low users	Psychotherapy users vs. Low users	Chiropractic & massage users vs. Low users	Mindfulness & relaxation users vs. Low users	High use multimodal vs. Low users
Female	0.08 (−0.03 to 0.18)	0.04 (−0.04 to 0.13)	0.16 (0.05 to 0.26)	0.03 (−0.05 to 0.11)	0.25 (0.16 to 0.35)
4 year degree	0.14 (0.08 to 0.19)	0.01 (−0.03 to 0.05)	0.09 (0.04 to 0.14)	0.09 (0.05 to 0.13)	0.07 (0.04 to 0.11)
Injured during deployment	0.02 (−0.04 to 0.09)	0.05 (0.01 to 0.09)	0.04 (−0.02 to 0.09)	−0.02 (−0.06 to 0.03)	0.06 (0.02 to 0.10)
Chronic Pain	0.03 (−0.03 to 0.09)	0.01 (−0.04 to 0.05)	0.15 (0.10 to 0.21)	−0.02 (−0.07 to 0.02)	0.06 (0.03 to 0.10)
Self-rated health Excellent/Very Good	0.12 (0.06 to 0.18)	−0.03 (−0.07 to 0.02)	0.04 (−0.01 to 0.10)	0.05 (0.00 to 0.09)	0.01 (−0.03 to 0.05)
Moderate or greater anxiety	0.03 (−0.06 to 0.12)	0.11 (0.05 to 0.17)	0.03 (−0.05 to 0.10)	0.07 (−0.01 to 0.15)	0.07 (0.01 to 0.13)
Depression	−0.05 (−0.14 to 0.03)	−0.01 (−0.05 to 0.04)	0.05 (−0.03 to 0.12)	−0.01 (−0.07 to 0.05)	−0.03 (−0.07 to 0.01)
PTSD	−0.03 (−0.13 to 0.06)	0.07 (0.01 to 0.13)	−0.03 (−0.10 to 0.05)	−0.02 (−0.08 to 0.05)	0.01 (−0.05 to 0.06)
Problem alcohol use	0.03 (−0.03 to 0.10)	−0.01 (−0.04 to 0.03)	−0.08 (−0.13 to −0.03)	−0.02 (−0.07 to 0.03)	0.02 (−0.02 to 0.06)
Any illicit drug use	0.00 (−0.09 to 0.09)	0.03 (−0.03 to 0.09)	0.13 (0.04 to 0.22)	0.13 (0.04 to 0.22)	−0.03 (−0.08 to 0.01)
Absorption †	0.08 (0.04 to 0.12)	0.03 (0.00 to 0.05)	0.02 (−0.01 to 0.06)	0.08 (0.05 to 0.11)	0.06 (0.04 to 0.08)

M: DISCUSSION AND SUMMARY

This dissertation had three main aims: 1) estimate the association of yoga and pain interference; 2) describe and explain similarities and differences in the yoga practice of those with chronic pain and those without chronic pain; and 3) explore how yoga fits into patterns of use of other health practices.

M.1. Summary of results

In Manuscript 1 ("Cross-sectional association of yoga..."), I estimated the association of yoga practice and pain interference (the degres to which pain interferes with life or causes disability). I used propensity score matching to control for potential confounding between yoga and interfering pain. I found that yoga practice is not associated with pain interference among veterans with pain. Yoga practitioners were quite similar to non-yoga practitioners, with notable differences being more women, higher educational attainment, slightly higher substance use and anxiety, and higher absorption. Propensity score matching was successful at balancing the differences between the two groups. I estimated the difference in prevalence of high interference pain in the two matched groups and calculated a 95% Confidence Interval. These results did not provide evidence for any association between yoga practice and pain interference. The results of the propensity score matched analysis were the same as results of a standard multivariable logistic regression and regression with yoga operationalized as multiple levels of frequency, showing the main results were robust to several methodological choices. Yoga practice has been shown to be beneficial at reducing pain and pain interference in randomized trials. The present results are potentially different for several reasons. First, because this was cross-sectional, people are in different time courses of yoga exposure and pain recovery, so there may be overlapping trends. Second, since yoga practice was self-reported, it did not have the same meaning across the exposure group. It is possible that the variety of meaning of yoga in the exposure group hides a true association. Finally, there may truly be no association between yoga and pain interference among a group of otherwise healthy people who self-select to yoga primarily for reasons other than pain. These findings highlight the importance of better understanding the variety of practices that a self-reported sample of yoga practitioners uses.

In Manuscript 2 ("How pain shapes the experience of yoga…"), I used a novel self-report instrument of yoga practice to examine for differences in yoga practice between people with chronic pain and people without chronic pain and examined possible explanations for those differences using qualitative interviews. I found that yoga practitioners with chronic pain report more self-directed practice rather than group instruction and less physically-challenging practices compared to yoga practitioners without chronic pain. In semi-structured interviews with yoga practitioners from the sample, it emerged that yoga practitioners with chronic pain feel self-conscious in group practice and therefore avoid them. Practitioners with chronic pain also expressed that they are frequently modifying (making less challenging or "backing off") their yoga practice within limitations they experience due to chronic pain. Yoga practitioners without chronic pain liked the social interactions and group dynamics of group practices. I successfully piloted a new self-report instrument of yoga practice, the Essential Properties of Yoga Questionnaire Short Form. Response rate was very good and missingness among respondents was low. This instrument should be investigated in other contexts. In particular, it would be very interesting to administer the instrument to yoga practitioners in the same or similar classes to see how their self-report is the same or different. If the EPYQ responses to similar yoga practices are quite different, it would suggest that individual factors and experiences have are important in practitioner perception of yoga practice. Also, it would be very interesting to administer the questionnaire to in a longitudinal study to examine the association of the different component sub-scales and improvements in pain.

In Manuscript 3 ("Patterns of use..."), I demonstrated the presence of six distinct classes of users of non-pharmacological health practices in a cohort of National Guard Veterans using latent class analysis. Approximately half of respondents use one or more of the 19 approaches of the Health Practices Inventory. They report that they are using practitioner-delivered approaches mostly for pain and active approaches for their general health and well-being. Active complementary approaches tended to cluster together in the use-patterns as did practitioner-delivered complementary approaches. Interestingly and relevant for the other studies in this dissertation, yoga appeared not to fit well as either practitioner-delivered or active. Multinomial logistic regression demonstrated that membership in each of these latent classes was associated with a unique set of predictors, some of which were key at distinguishing the classes. The Psychotherapy users class had higher levels of distress. The

Exercise users class was in excellent overall health. Absorption was associated with classes that used active practices. Being female and having chronic pain was associated with use of practitioner-delivered complementary approaches. Additionally, I successfully administered a novel instrument to self-report integrated use of active and practitioner-delivered complementary and conventional approaches for health reasons. The Health Practices Inventory is ready to be used by other investigators as a standardized way to measure and report on use of non-pharmacological therapies in their studies.

M.2. Conceptual models

I was not able to fully test the models that I presented earlier ("Effect of yoga on pain interference," p. 12, and "Relationship between mode and maintenance of yoga practice," p. 18), but I did learn about some key relationships depicted in the models.

In Manuscript 2 ("How pain shapes the experience of yoga…"), I observed that continuing yoga practitioners (people that were still using yoga a year after their first report) had a lower prevalence of chronic pain and higher self-rated health compared to discontinued yoga practitioners. An important next step would be to see if those observed differences between maintained and discontinued yoga practitioners in the follow-up survey are due to baseline differences or change over time. If the observed differences are due to change over time, that would support the portion of my model that links perceived benefits to maintenance of practice. The number of discontinued yoga practitioners was very small in this study and only very large effects would be detectable statistically.

In Manuscript 1 ("Cross-sectional association..."), I observed that mental health vulnerability was associated with high interference pain (Table J-2, p. 53), but not yoga practice (Table J-3, p. 54). More open and mindful personality (absorption) was associated both with higher pain interference and yoga practice. An important follow-up study would be to look at the association of these variables and initiation of yoga practice. Ultimately, yoga practice was not associated with pain interference, both in crude, unadjusted regression, and adjusted, propensity score-matched analysis. These dual, lack of associations are hard to interpret (as described above), but I would hypothesize one reason for the lack of association is because there is one large group of yoga practitioners that is doing quite well and another group that struggles with their health and uses yoga to improve their health. Additionally, yoga practitioners may initially adopt yoga for pain, then switch their reason for maintaining a yoga practice to general wellness when their pain improves. This changing reason would be consistent with other findings that motivations for practicing yoga shift between from initiation and maintenance.[170]

Manuscript 3 ("Patterns of use...") shows a hint of the multiple classes of yoga practitioners. First of all, it is very clear that yoga practitioners are using numerous other health practices (Table L-4, p. 116). An important number of yoga practitioners are very highly engaged with other health practices. Second, most yoga practitioners were actually in the exercise latent class. Similar to maintained yoga practitioners, the exercise class was associated with better self-rated health. Both of these findings are consistent with stated reason for use of yoga (Table L-1, p. 112), which shows that a vast majority of yoga practitioners use yoga for their general health. Finally, the highest health practice utilizing yoga practitioners belong to the multimodal class, which is also associated with higher chronic pain. The yoga practitioners with chronic pain practice yoga differently and express feelings of self-consciousness in group practice, which is a barrier and leads them to practice independently.

The next steps to test the models would be longitudinal studies that test the relationship of baseline characteristics with adoption of yoga practice, yoga practice with changing characteristics, changed characteristics with maintenance of practice, and maintained yoga practice with pain vulnerability/resilience factors. A longitudinal study of the role of pain resilience/vulnerability factors in changing pain disability would not need to be restricted to yoga practitioners but would be a critical piece in understanding the model. Figure M-1 (p. 131) presents an updated, integrated model of the study, showing next steps.

M.3. Discussion

Overall, this dissertation makes several contributions to general knowledge about yoga and use of other non-pharmacological therapies. Despite evidence for its effectiveness in pain, people are generally using yoga for reasons other than pain. When people with chronic pain do use yoga, they are practicing in a different way than their counterparts without chronic pain. I have made two new instruments available to aid further exploration of this topic. The self-report version of the Essential Properties of Yoga Questionnaire could allow for investigation into what components of yoga practices are important for pain management. This tool could be clinically useful in designing integrated pain treatments. Investigators should pay attention to the specific barriers and facilitators to yoga practice that people with pain experience and ensure that study participants are not limited to group practices. Further evidence is needed as to the effectiveness of self-directed practices versus group instruction and how to deliver them effectively. Second, the Health Practices Inventory allows broad exploration of how people are using many non-pharmacological therapies in an integrated fashion, because as was seen, a majority of people are using non-pharmacological therapies, and a majority of them are using multiple approaches together.

    This dissertation is a beginning of an exploration into how yoga practitioners are using yoga and what parts of their practice are beneficial. The way people use yoga in the "real world" is akin to intervention fidelity. When clinicians recommend yoga practice as part of a multimodal pain treatment plan, does it matter what kind of yoga they do? This dissertation provides some important information about tools that I can use in this further exploration and hints of differences in practice I can expect to observe. Also, the models I developed for the dissertation provide important next steps and show important studies to perform. A better understanding of the unified conceptual model would bring important contributions to pain research and care as well as optimization of yoga and related health practices. As I move forward in my research and clinical career, I will strive towards these contributions and to provide evidence-based integrative care to my future patients.

Figure M-1: Updated, integrated conceptual model of this dissertation, with next steps numbered

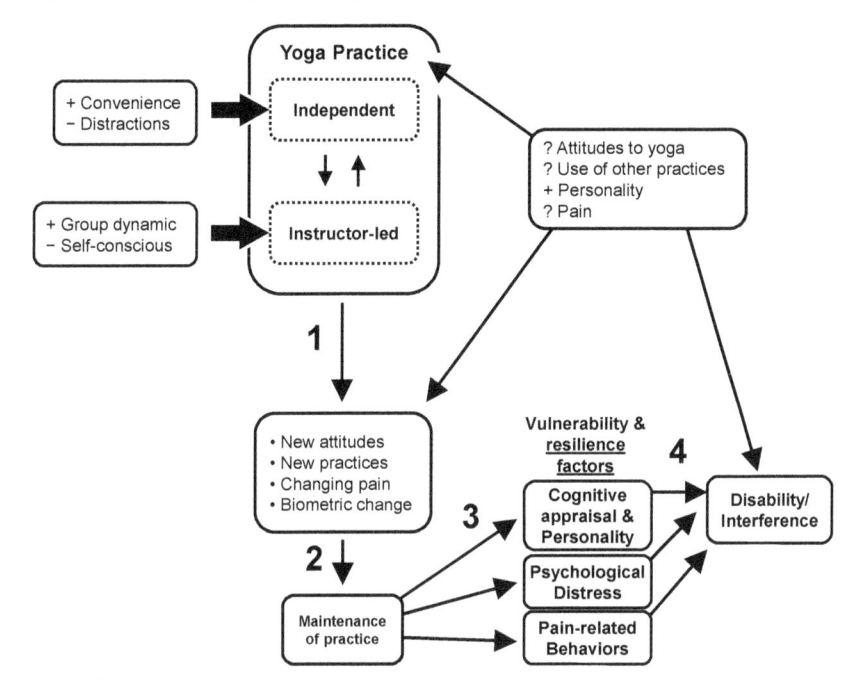

N: BIBLIOGRAPHY

1. IOM (Institute of Medicine). *Relieving Pain in America: A Blueprint for Transforming Prevention, Care, Education, and Research.* Washington, DC; 2011. http://www.nap.edu/catalog.php?record_id=13172.

2. Abajobir AA, Abate KH, Abbafati C, et al. Global, regional, and national disability-adjusted life-years (DALYs) for 333 diseases and injuries and healthy life expectancy (HALE) for 195 countries and territories, 1990–2016: a systematic analysis for the Global Burden of Disease Study 2016. *Lancet.* 2017;390(10100):1260-1344. doi:10.1016/S0140-6736(17)32130-X

3. Mokdad AH, Ballestros K, Echko M, et al. The State of US Health, 1990-2016. *JAMA.* 2018;319(14):1444. doi:10.1001/jama.2018.0158

4. Hoy D, March L, Brooks P, et al. The global burden of low back pain: estimates from the Global Burden of Disease 2010 study. *Ann Rheum Dis.* 2014;73(6):968-974. doi:10.1136/annrheumdis-2013-204428

5. Mafi JN, McCarthy EP, Davis RB, Landon BE. Worsening trends in the management and treatment of back pain. *JAMA Intern Med.* 2013;173(17):1573. doi:10.1001/jamainternmed.2013.8992

6. Clark ME. Post-deployment pain: A need for rapid detection and intervention. *Pain Med.* 2004;5(4):333-334. doi:10.1111/j.1526-4637.2004.04059.x

7. Haskell SG, Brandt CA, Krebs EE, Skanderson M, Kerns RD, Goulet JL. Pain among veterans of operations enduring freedom and Iraqi Freedom: Do women and men differ? *Pain Med.* 2009;10(7):1167-1173. doi:10.1111/j.1526-4637.2009.00714.x

8. Kazis LE, Miller DR, Clark J, et al. Health-Related Quality of Life in Patients Served by the Department of Veterans Affairs. *Arch Intern Med.* 1998;158(6):626. doi:10.1001/archinte.158.6.626

9. Haskell SG, Heapy A, Reid MC, Papas RK, Kerns RD. The prevalence and age-related characteristics of pain in a sample of women veterans receiving primary care. *J Womens Health (Larchmt).* 2006;15(7):862-869. doi:10.1089/jwh.2006.15.862

10. Pham HH, Schrag D, Hargraves JL, Bach PB. Delivery of preventive services to older adults by primary care physicians. *JAMA J Am Med Assoc.* 2005;294(4):473-481. doi:10.1111/j.1365-4632.2008.03871.x

11. Kerns RD, Otis J, Rosenberg R, Reid MC. Veterans' reports of pain and associations with ratings of health, health-risk behaviors, affective distress, and use of the healthcare system. *J Rehabil Res Dev.* 2003;40(5):371-379. doi:10.1682/JRRD.2003.09.0371

12. Last AR, Hulbert K. Chronic lower back pain. *Am Fam Physician.* 2009;79(12):1067-1074. doi:10.1007/s00115-011-3421-5

13. Chou R, Qaseem A, Snow V, et al. Diagnosis and treatment of low back pain: A joint clinical practice guideline from the American College of Physicians and the American Pain Society. *Ann Intern Med.* 2007;147(July):478-491. doi:10.7326/0003-4819-147-7-200710020-00006
14. Dowell D, Haegerich TM, Chou R. CDC Guideline for Prescribing Opioids for Chronic Pain — United States, 2016. *MMWR Recomm Reports.* 2016;65(1):1-49. doi:10.15585/mmwr.rr6501e1
15. Tarphon R. Classification of chronic pain. Descriptions of chronic pain syndromes and definitions of pain terms. Prepared by the International Association for the Study of Pain, Subcommittee on Taxonomy. *Pain Suppl.* 1986;3:S1-226. http://www.ncbi.nlm.nih.gov/pubmed/3461421.
16. Von Korff M, Ormel J, Keefe FJ, Dworkin SF. Grading the severity of chronic pain. *Pain.* 1992;50(2):133-149. doi:10.1016/0304-3959(92)90154-4
17. van Tulder MW, Scholten RJPM, Koes BW, Deyo RA. Nonsteroidal Anti-Inflammatory Drugs for Low Back Pain. *Spine (Phila Pa 1976).* 2000;25(19):2501-2513. doi:10.1097/00007632-200010010-00013
18. Urquhart DM, Hoving JL, Assendelft WJ, Roland M, van Tulder MW. Antidepressants for non-specific low back pain. *Cochrane Database Syst Rev.* 2008;1(1):CD001703. doi:10.1002/14651858.CD001703.pub3
19. Van Tulder M, Touray T, Furlan A, Solway S, Bouter L. Muscle relaxants for non-specific low-back pain (Review). *Cochrane Collab.* 2008;(4). doi:10.1002/14651858.CD004252.
20. Chaparro LE, Furlan AD, Deshpande A, Mailis-Gagnon A, Atlas S, Turk DC. Opioids compared to placebo or other treatments for chronic low-back pain. *Cochrane Database Syst Rev.* 2013;8(8):CD004959. doi:10.1002/14651858.CD004959.pub4
21. Mathieson S, Kasch R, Maher CG, et al. Combination drug therapy for low back pain. *Cochrane Database Syst Rev.* 2015;(12). doi:10.1002/14651858.CD011982
22. Krebs EE, Paudel M, Taylor BC, et al. Association of Opioids with Falls, Fractures, and Physical Performance among Older Men with Persistent Musculoskeletal Pain. *J Gen Intern Med.* 2016;31(5):463-469. doi:10.1007/s11606-015-3579-9
23. Gaither JR, Goulet JL, Becker WC, et al. The Association Between Receipt of Guideline-Concordant Long-Term Opioid Therapy and All-Cause Mortality. *J Gen Intern Med.* 2016;31(5):492-501. doi:10.1007/s11606-015-3571-4
24. Morasco BJ, Yarborough BJ, Smith NX, et al. Higher Prescription Opioid Dose is Associated With Worse Patient-Reported Pain Outcomes and More Health Care Utilization. *J Pain.* 2017;18(4):437-445.

doi:10.1016/j.jpain.2016.12.004

25. Krebs EE, Gravely A, Nugent S, et al. Effect of opioid vs nonopioid medications on pain-related function in patients with chronic back pain or hip or knee osteoarthritis pain the SPACE randomized clinical trial. *JAMA - J Am Med Assoc.* 2018;319(9):872-882. doi:10.1001/jama.2018.0899

26. Geneen L, Smith B, Clarke C, Martin D, Colvin LA, Moore RA. Physical activity and exercise for chronic pain in adults: an overview of Cochrane reviews. *Cochrane Database Syst Rev.* 2014;(2014 Issue 8):11279. doi:10.1002/14651858.CD011279

27. Office of the Army Surgeon General. Pain Management Task Force Final Report. http://www.health.mil/Reference-Center/Presentations/2010/06/08/Defense-and-Veterans-Pain-Management-Initiative. Published 2010. Accessed February 2, 2018.

28. Krebs EE, Kerns RD. Meeting the challenge of chronic pain as a public health problem. FORUM. http://www.hsrd.research.va.gov/publications/forum/spring16/default.cfm. Published 2016.

29. Glicken MD. *Learning from Resilient People: Lessons We Can Apply to Counseling and Psychotherapy.* Thousand Oaks, CA: Sage Publications; 2006.

30. Sturgeon JA, Zautra AJ. Resilience: A new paradigm for adaptation to chronic pain. *Curr Pain Headache Rep.* 2010;14(2):105-112. doi:10.1007/s11916-010-0095-9

31. Prince-Embury S, Saklofske D, eds. *Resilience in Children, Adolescents, and Adults: Translating Research into Practice.* Springer New York; 2013. doi:10.1007/978-1-4614-4939-3

32. Taylor S, MacArthur Foundation Psychosocial Working Group. Psychosocial Notebook: Coping Strategies. http://www.macses.ucsf.edu/research/psychosocial/coping.php. Accessed April 4, 2015.

33. Lazarus RS. Toward better research on stress and coping. *Am Psychol.* 2000;55(6):665-673. doi:10.1037/0003-066X.55.6.665

34. Rippetoe P a, Rogers RW. Effects of components of protection-motivation theory on adaptive and maladaptive coping with a health threat. *J Pers Soc Psychol.* 1987;52(3):596-604. doi:10.1037/0022-3514.52.3.596

35. Wadsworth ME. Development of Maladaptive Coping: A Functional Adaptation to Chronic, Uncontrollable Stress. *Child Dev Perspect.* 2015;9(2):96-100. doi:10.1111/cdep.12112

36. Leeuw M, Goossens MEJB, Linton SJ, Crombez G, Boersma K, Vlaeyen JWS. The fear-avoidance model of musculoskeletal pain: Current state of scientific evidence. *J Behav Med.* 2007;30(1):77-94. doi:10.1007/s10865-

006-9085-0

37. Wong PTP, Wong LCJ, eds. *Handbook of Multicultural Perspectives on Stress and Coping.* Springer New York; 2006. doi:10.1007/b137168
38. Lazarus RS, DeLongis A. Psychological stress and coping in aging. *Am Psychol.* 1983;38(3):245-254. doi:10.2190/T43T-84P3-QDUR-7RTP
39. Denk F, McMahon SB, Tracey I. Pain vulnerability: a neurobiological perspective. *Nat Neurosci.* 2014;17(2):192-200. doi:10.1038/nn.3628
40. Reich JW, Zautra AJ, Hall JS. *Handbook of Adult Resilience.* New York: Guilford Press; 2010.
41. Cramer H, Lauche R, Haller H, Dobos G. A systematic review and meta-analysis of yoga for low back pain. *Clin J Pain.* 2013;29(5):450-460. doi:10.1097/AJP.0b013e31825e1492
42. McCall T. *Yoga As Medicine: The Yogic Prescription for Health and Healing.* New York, New York: Bantam Dell; 2007.
43. Mitchell J, Trangle M, Degnan B, et al. *Adult Depression in Primary Care.* Bloomington, MN; 2013. https://www.guideline.gov/content.aspx?id=47315.
44. Diagnosis and Management of Hypertension Working Group. VA/DoD clinical practice guideline for the diagnosis and management of hypertension in the primary care setting. 2014:135. https://www.guideline.gov/content.aspx?id=48858&search=yoga+and+hypertension.
45. Cramer H, Ward L, Steel A, Lauche R, Dobos G, Zhang Y. Prevalence, Patterns, and Predictors of Yoga Use: Results of a U.S. Nationally Representative Survey. *Am J Prev Med.* 2016;50(2):230-235. doi:10.1016/j.amepre.2015.07.037
46. Verrastro G. Yoga as therapy. *J Fam Pract.* 2014;63(9):E1-E6. http://www.jfponline.com/fileadmin/qhi/jfp/pdfs/6309/JFP_06309_ArticleW1.pdf.
47. Birdee GS, Legedza AT, Saper RB, Bertisch SM, Eisenberg DM, Phillips RS. Characteristics of Yoga Users: Results of a National Survey. *J Gen Intern Med.* 2008;23(10):1653-1658. doi:10.1007/s11606-008-0735-5
48. Park CL, Braun T, Siegel T. Who practices yoga? A systematic review of demographic, health-related, and psychosocial factors associated with yoga practice. *J Behav Med.* 2015. doi:10.1007/s10865-015-9618-5
49. Cramer H, Lauche R, Langhorst J, Paul A, Michalsen A, Dobos G. Predictors of yoga use among internal medicine patients. *BMC Complement Altern Med.* 2013;13(1):172. doi:10.1186/1472-6882-13-172
50. Salmon P, Lush E, Jablonski M, Sephton SE. Yoga and Mindfulness: Clinical Aspects of an Ancient Mind/Body Practice. *Cogn Behav Pract.* 2009;16(1):59-72. doi:10.1016/j.cbpra.2008.07.002

51. Genovese JEC, Fondran KM. The Psychology of Yoga Practitioners: A Cluster Analysis. *Int J Yoga Therap*. 2017;27(1):51-58. doi:10.17761/1531-2054-27.1.51
52. Singleton M. *Yoga Body: The Origins of Modern Posture Practice*. New York, NY: Oxford University Press; 2010.
53. De Michelis E. *A History of Modern Yoga: Patanjali and Western Esotericism*. London: Continuum; 2005.
54. Cramer H, Lauche R, Langhorst J, Dobos G. Is one yoga style better than another? A systematic review of associations of yoga style and conclusions in randomized yoga trials. *Complement Ther Med*. 2016;25(2016):178-187. doi:10.1016/j.ctim.2016.02.015
55. Sherman KJ. Guidelines for developing yoga interventions for randomized trials. *Evidence-Based Complement Altern Med*. 2012;2012:1-16. doi:10.1155/2012/143271
56. Ward L, Stebbings S, Cherkin D, Baxter GD. Components and reporting of yoga interventions for musculoskeletal conditions: A systematic review of randomised controlled trials. *Complement Ther Med*. 2014;22(5):909-919. doi:10.1016/j.ctim.2014.08.007
57. Ward L, Stebbings S, Sherman KJ, Cherkin D, Baxter GD. Establishing key components of yoga interventions for musculoskeletal conditions: a Delphi survey. *BMC Complement Altern Med*. 2014;14(1):196. doi:10.1186/1472-6882-14-196
58. de Manincor M, Bensoussan A, Smith C, Fahey P, Bourchier S. Establishing key components of yoga interventions for reducing depression and anxiety, and improving well-being: a Delphi method study. *BMC Complement Altern Med*. 2015;15(1):1-10. doi:10.1186/s12906-015-0614-7
59. Broad WJ. *The Science of Yoga: The Risks and the Rewards*. 1st ed. New York: Simon & Schuster; 2012.
60. Schmalzl L, Streeter C, Khalsa S. Research on the psychophysiology of yoga. In: Khalsa S, Cohen L, McCall T, Telles S, eds. *The Principles and Practice of Yoga in Health Care*. Edinburgh, UK: Handspring Publishing; 2016:49-70.
61. Kinser PA, Goehler LE, Taylor AG. How might yoga help depression. *Explor J Sci Heal*. 2012;8(2):118-126. doi:10.1016/j.explore.2011.12.005
62. Gard T, Noggle JJ, Park CL, Vago DR, Wilson A. Potential self-regulatory mechanisms of yoga for psychological health. *Front Hum Neurosci*. 2014;8(September):1-20. doi:10.3389/fnhum.2014.00770
63. Hallman DM, Lyskov E. Autonomic Regulation in Musculoskeletal Pain. In: *Pain in Perspective*. InTech Open; 2012. doi:10.5772/51086
64. Buckenmaier CI, Schoomaker E. Patients ' Use of Active Self-Care

Complementary and Integrative Medicine in Their Management of Chronic Pain Symptoms. 2014:7-8.

65. Crawford C, Lee C, Buckenmaier C, Schoomaker E, Petri R, Jonas W. The Current State of the Science for Active Self-Care Complementary and Integrative Medicine Therapies in the Management of Chronic Pain Symptoms: Lessons Learned, Directions for the Future. *Pain Med.* 2014;15(S1):S104-S113. doi:10.1111/pme.12406

66. Meng X-G, Yue S-W. Efficacy of aerobic exercise for treatment of chronic low back pain. *Am J Phys Med Rehabil.* 2015;94(5):358-365. doi:10.1097/PHM.0000000000000188

67. Ferreira ML, Smeets RJEM, Kamper SJ, Ferreira PH, Machado LAC. Can we explain heterogeneity among randomized clinical trials of exercise for chronic back pain? A meta-regression analysis of randomized controlled trials. *Phys Ther.* 2010;90(10):1383-1403. doi:10.2522/ptj.20090332

68. Gatchel RJ, Rollings KH. Evidence-informed management of chronic low back pain with cognitive behavioral therapy. *Spine J.* 2008;8(1):40-44. doi:10.1016/j.spinee.2007.10.007

69. Sherman KJ, Cherkin DC, Erro J, Miglioretti DL, Deyo RA. Comparing yoga, exercise, and a self-care book for chronic low back pain: A randomized, controlled trial. *Ann Intern Med.* 2005;143(12):849-856. doi:10.1016/S0084-3873(08)70341-9

70. Sherman KJ, Cherkin DC, Wellman RD, et al. A randomized trial comparing yoga, stretching, and a self-care book for chronic low back pain. *Arch Intern Med.* 2011;171(22):2019-2026. doi:10.1001/archinternmed.2011.524

71. Sherman KJ, Cherkin DC, Cook AJ, et al. Comparison of yoga versus stretching for chronic low back pain: protocol for the Yoga Exercise Self-care (YES) trial. *Trials.* 2010;11(1):36. doi:10.1186/1745-6215-11-36

72. Sherman KJ, Wellman RD, Cook AJ, Cherkin DC, Ceballos RM. Mediators of yoga and stretching for chronic low back pain. *Evidence-Based Complement Altern Med.* 2013;2013:1-11. doi:10.1155/2013/130818

73. Park CL, Elwy AR, Maiya M, et al. The Essential Properties of Yoga Questionnaire (EPYQ): Psychometric Properties. *Int J Yoga Therap.* March 2018:epub ahead of print. doi:10.17761/2018-00016R2

74. Amtmann D, Cook KF, Jensen MP, et al. Development of a PROMIS item bank to measure pain interference. *Pain.* 2010;150(1):173-182. doi:10.1016/j.pain.2010.04.025

75. Yeung EW, Arewasikporn A, Zautra AJ. Resilience and Chronic Pain. *J Soc Clin Psychol.* 2012;31(6):593-617. doi:10.1521/jscp.2012.31.6.593

76. Saltychev M, Bärlund E, Laimi K. Correlation between the pain numeric rating scale and the 12-item WHO Disability Assessment Schedule 2.0 in

patients with musculoskeletal pain. *Int J Rehabil Res.* 2018;41(1):87-91. doi:10.1097/MRR.0000000000000262

77. Kanodia AK, Legedza ATR, Davis RB, Eisenberg DM, Phillips RS. Perceived benefit of complementary and alternative medicine (CAM) for back pain: A national survey. *J Am Board Fam Med.* 2010;23(3):354-362. doi:10.3122/jabfm.2010.03.080252

78. Saper RB, Eisenberg DM, Davis RB, Culpepper L, Phillips RS. Prevalence and patterns of adult yoga use in the United States: Results of a national survey. *Altern Ther Health Med.* 2004;10(2):44-49.

79. Coeytaux R, McDuffie J, Goode A, et al. *Evidence Map of Yoga for High-Impact Conditions Affecting Veterans.* VA ESP Project #09-010; 2014.

80. Lakke SE, Soer R, Takken T, Reneman MF. Risk and prognostic factors for non-specific musculoskeletal pain: A synthesis of evidence from systematic reviews classified into ICF dimensions. *Pain.* 2009;147(1-3):153-164. doi:10.1016/j.pain.2009.08.032

81. Martz E, Livneh H. *Coping with Chronic Illness and Disability.* (Martz E, Livneh H, eds.). Boston, MA: Springer US; 2007. doi:10.1007/978-0-387-48670-3

82. Fish RA, McGuire B, Hogan M, Morrison TG, Stewart I. Validation of the Chronic Pain Acceptance Questionnaire (CPAQ) in an Internet sample and development and preliminary validation of the CPAQ-8. *Pain.* 2010;149(3):435-443. doi:10.1016/j.pain.2009.12.016

83. Hirsh AT, George SZ, Riley JL, Robinson ME. An evaluation of the measurement of pain catastrophizing by the coping strategies questionnaire. *Eur J Pain.* 2007;11(1):75-75. doi:10.1016/j.ejpain.2005.12.010

84. Hibbard JH, Mahoney ER, Stockard J, Tusler M. Development and testing of a short form of the patient activation measure. *Health Serv Res.* 2005;40(6p1):1918-1930. doi:10.1111/j.1475-6773.2005.00438.x

85. Bendayan R, Esteve R, Blanca MJ. New empirical evidence of the validity of the Chronic Pain Acceptance Questionnaire: The differential influence of activity engagement and pain willingness on adjustment to chronic pain. *Br J Health Psychol.* 2012;17(2):314-326. doi:10.1111/j.2044-8287.2011.02039.x

86. Arnow B a., Blasey CM, Constantino MJ, et al. Catastrophizing, depression and pain-related disability. *Gen Hosp Psychiatry.* 2011;33(2):150-156. doi:10.1016/j.genhosppsych.2010.12.008

87. Kroenke K, Strine TW, Spitzer RL, Williams JBW, Berry JT, Mokdad AH. The PHQ-8 as a measure of current depression in the general population. *J Affect Disord.* 2009;114(1-3):163-173. doi:10.1016/j.jad.2008.06.026

88. Blanchard EB, Jones-Alexander J, Buckley TC, Forneris CA. Psychometric

properties of the PTSD checklist (PCL). *Behav Res Ther.* 1996;34(8):669-673. doi:10.1016/0005-7967(96)00033-2

89. Chou R, Shekelle P. Will this patient develop persistent disabling low back pain? *JAMA.* 2010;303(13):1295. doi:10.1001/jama.2010.344

90. Skinner HA. The drug abuse screening test. *Addict Behav.* 1982;7(4):363-371. doi:10.1016/0306-4603(82)90005-3

91. Meneses-Gaya C, Zuardi AW, Loureiro SR, et al. Is the full version of the AUDIT really necessary? Study of the validity and internal construct of tts abbreviated versions. *Alcohol Clin Exp Res.* 2010;34(8):no-no. doi:10.1111/j.1530-0277.2010.01225.x

92. Morasco BJ, Corson K, Turk DC, Dobscha SK. Association between substance use disorder status and pain-related function following 12 months of treatment in primary care patients with musculoskeletal pain. *J Pain.* 2011;12(3):352-359. doi:10.1016/j.jpain.2010.07.010

93. Villemure C, Ceko M, Cotton V a, Bushnell MC. Insular cortex mediates increased pain tolerance in yoga practitioners. *Cereb Cortex.* 2013;(October):1-9. doi:10.1093/cercor/bht124

94. Shapiro D, Cook I a., Davydov DM, Ottaviani C, Leuchter AF, Abrams M. Yoga as a complementary treatment of depression: Effects of traits and moods on treatment outcome. *Evidence-based Complement Altern Med.* 2007;4(4):493-502. doi:10.1093/ecam/nel114

95. Saper RB, Sherman KJ, Cullum-Dugan D, Davis RB, Phillips RS, Culpepper L. Yoga for chronic low back pain in a predominantly minority population: a pilot randomized controlled trial. *Altern Ther Health Med.* 2009;15(6):18-27.

96. Combs MA, Thorn BE. Yoga attitudes in chronic low back pain: Roles of catastrophizing and fear of movement. *Complement Ther Clin Pract.* 2015;21(3):160-165. doi:10.1016/j.ctcp.2015.06.006

97. Schütze R, Rees C, Preece M, Schütze M. Low mindfulness predicts pain catastrophizing in a fear-avoidance model of chronic pain. *Pain.* 2010;148(1):120-127. doi:10.1016/j.pain.2009.10.030

98. Curtis K, Osadchuk A, Katz J. An eight-week yoga intervention is associated with improvements in pain, psychological functioning and mindfulness, and changes in cortisol levels in women with fibromyalgia. *J Pain Res.* 2011;4:189-201. doi:10.2147/JPR.S22761

99. Belle I, Handler L, Guthmann R. Can yoga reduce symptoms of anxiety and depression? *J Fam Pract.* 2014;63(7):398-407.

100. Keosaian JE, Lemaster CM, Dresner D, et al. "We're all in this together": A qualitative study of predominantly low income minority participants in a yoga trial for chronic low back pain. *Complement Ther Med.* 2016;24:34-39. doi:10.1016/j.ctim.2015.11.007

101. Saper RB, Boah AR, Keosaian J, Cerrada C, Weinberg J, Sherman KJ. Comparing once-versus twice-weekly yoga classes for chronic low back pain in predominantly low income minorities: A randomized dosing trial. *Evidence-based Complement Altern Med.* 2013;2013. doi:10.1155/2013/658030

102. Spadola CE, Rottapel R, Khandpur N, et al. Enhancing yoga participation: A qualitative investigation of barriers and facilitators to yoga among predominantly racial/ethnic minority, low-income adults. *Complement Ther Clin Pract.* 2017;29:97-104. doi:10.1016/j.ctcp.2017.09.001

103. Blevins CA, Weathers FW, Davis MT, Witte TK, Domino JL. The Posttraumatic Stress Disorder Checklist for DSM-5 (PCL-5): Development and initial psychometric evaluation. *J Trauma Stress.* 2015;28(6):489-498. doi:10.1002/jts.22059

104. Patrick CJ, Curtin JJ, Tellegen A. Development and validation of a brief form of the Multidimensional Personality Questionnaire. *Psychol Assess.* 2002;14(2):150-163. doi:10.1037/1040-3590.14.2.150

105. Damush TMM, Kroenke K, Bair MJJ, et al. Pain self-management training increases self-efficacy, self-management behaviours and pain and depression outcomes. *Eur J Pain (United Kingdom).* 2016;20(7):1070-1078. doi:10.1002/ejp.830

106. Tunks ER, Crook J, Weir R. Epidemiology of chronic pain with psychological comorbidity: Prevalence, risk, course, and prognosis. *La Rev Can Psychiatr.* 2008;53(4):224-234.

107. Bair MJ, Robinson RL, Katon W, Kroenke K. Depression and Pain Comorbidity. *Arch Intern Med.* 2003;163(20):2433. doi:10.1001/archinte.163.20.2433

108. Ang DC, Outcalt SD, Wu J, Sargent C, Yu Z, Bair MJ. Pain experience of Iraq and Afghanistan Veterans with comorbid chronic pain and posttraumatic stress. *J Rehabil Res Dev.* 2014;51(4):559-570 12p. doi:10.1682/JRRD.2013.06.0134

109. Spitzer RL, Kroenke K, Williams JBW, PHQ-PCS. Validation and Utility of a Self-report Version of PRIME-MD. *JAMA J Am Med Assoc.* 1999;282(18):1737-1744. doi:10.1001/jama.282.18.1737

110. Kroenke K, Spitzer RL, Williams JBW. The PHQ-9: Validity of a brief depression severity measure. *J Gen Intern Med.* 2001;16(9):606-613. doi:10.1046/j.1525-1497.2001.016009606.x

111. Löwe B, Unützer J, Callahan CM, Perkins AJ, Kroenke K. Monitoring depression treatment outcomes with the patient health questionnaire-9. *Med Care.* 2004;42(12):1194-1201. doi:10.1097/00005650-200412000-00006

112. Martin A, Rief W, Klaiberg A, Braehler E. Validity of the Brief Patient Health

Questionnaire Mood Scale (PHQ-9) in the general population. *Gen Hosp Psychiatry*. 2006;28(1):71-77. doi:10.1016/j.genhosppsych.2005.07.003

113. Pinto-Meza A, Serrano-Blanco A, Peñarrubia MT, Blanco E, Haro JM. Assessing depression in primary care with the PHQ-9: Can it be carried out over the telephone? *J Gen Intern Med*. 2005;20(8):738-742. doi:10.1111/j.1525-1497.2005.0144.x

114. Seal K, Metzler T, Gima K, Bertenthal D, Maguen S, Marmar C. Trends and risk factors for mental health diagnoses among Iraq and Afghanistan veterans using Department of Veterans Affairs health care, 2002-2008. *Am J Public Health*. 2009;99(9):1651-1658.

115. Meis L a., Erbes CR, Kaler ME, Arbisi P a., Polusny M a. The structure of PTSD among two cohorts of returning soldiers: Before, during, and following deployment to Iraq. *J Abnorm Psychol*. 2011;120(4):807-818. doi:10.1037/a0023976

116. Morasco BJ, Lovejoy TI, Lu M, Turk DC, Lewis L, Dobscha SK. The relationship between PTSD and chronic pain: Mediating role of coping strategies and depression. *Pain*. 2013;154(4):609-616. doi:10.1016/j.pain.2013.01.001

117. Seal KH, Shi Y, Cohen G, et al. Association of Mental Health Disorders With Prescription Opioids and High-Risk Opioid Use in US Veterans of Iraq and Afghanistan. *JAMA J Am Med Assoc*. 2012;307(9):940. doi:10.1001/jama.2012.234

118. Wortmann JH, Jordan AH, Weathers FW, et al. Psychometric Analysis of the PTSD Checklist-5 (PCL-5) Among Treatment-Seeking Military Service Members. *Psychol Assess*. 2016;5. doi:10.1037/pas0000260

119. Keen SM, Kutter CJ, Niles BL, Krinsley KE. Psychometric properties of PTSD Checklist in sample of male veterans. *J Rehabil Res Dev*. 2008;45(3):465-474. doi:10.1682/JRRD.2007.09.0138

120. Bovin MJ, Marx BP, Weathers FW, et al. Psychometric properties of the PTSD checklist for diagnostic and statistical manual of mental disorders-fifth edition (PCL-5) in veterans. *Psychol Assess*. 2016;5(11):0-13. doi:10.1037/pas0000254

121. Seal KH, Cohen G, Waldrop A, Cohen BE, Maguen S, Ren L. Substance use disorders in Iraq and Afghanistan veterans in VA healthcare, 2001-2010: Implications for screening, diagnosis and treatment. *Drug Alcohol Depend*. 2011;116(1-3):93-101. doi:10.1016/j.drugalcdep.2010.11.027

122. McCabe SE, Boyd CJ, Cranford JA, Morales M, Slayden J. A modified version of the Drug Abuse Screening Test among undergraduate students. *J Subst Abuse Treat*. 2006;31(3):297-303. doi:10.1016/j.jsat.2006.04.010

123. Carey KB, Cocco KM, Simons JS. Concurrent validity of clinicians' ratings of substance abuse among psychiatric outpatients. *Psychiatr Serv*.

1996;47(8):842-847. doi:10.1176/ps.47.8.842

124. Carey MP, Morrison-Beedy D, Carey KB, Maisto SA, Gordon CM, Pedlow CT. Psychiatric outpatients report their experiences as participants in a randomized clinical trial. *J Nerv Ment Dis.* 2001;189(5):299-306. http://www.ncbi.nlm.nih.gov/pubmed/11379973.

125. Skinner HA, Goldberg AE. Evidence for a drug dependence syndrome among narcotic users. *Br J Addict.* 1986;81(4):479-484. doi:10.1111/j.1360-0443.1986.tb00359.x

126. Gavin DR, Ross HE, Skinner HA. Diagnostic validity of the drug abuse screening test in the assessment of DSM-III drug disorders. *Br J Addict.* 1989;84(3):301-307. doi:10.1111/j.1360-0443.1989.tb03463.x

127. Helmer DA, Chandler HK, Quigley KS, Blatt M, Teichman R, Lange G. Chronic widespread pain, mental health, and physical role function in OEF/OIF veterans. *Pain Med.* 2009;10(7):1174-1182. doi:10.1111/j.1526-4637.2009.00723.x

128. Saunders JB, Aasland OG, Babor TF, De La Fuente JR, Grant M. Development of the Alcohol Use Disorders Identification Test (AUDIT): WHO collaborative project on early detection of persons with harmful alcohol consumption--II. *Addiction.* 1993;88(6):791-804. doi:10.1111/j.1360-0443.1993.tb02093.x

129. Tellegen A, Waller NG. Exploring Personality Through Test Construction: Development of the Multidimensional Personality Questionnaire. In: *The SAGE Handbook of Personality Theory and Assessment: Volume 2 — Personality Measurement and Testing.* 1 Oliver's Yard, 55 City Road, London EC1Y 1SP United Kingdom: SAGE Publications Ltd; :261-292. doi:10.4135/9781849200479.n13

130. Tellegen A, Atkinson G. Openness to absorbing and self-altering experiences ("absorption"), a trait related to hypnotic susceptibility. *J Abnorm Psychol.* 1974;83(3):268-277. http://www.ncbi.nlm.nih.gov/pubmed/4844914.

131. Watson D, Clark LA, Tellegen A. Development and validation of brief measures of positive and negative affect: the PANAS scales. *J Pers Soc Psychol.* 1988;54(6):1063-1070. doi:10.1037/0022-3514.54.6.1063

132. Galbraith N, Moss T, Galbraith V, Purewal S. A systematic review of the traits and cognitions associated with use of and belief in complementary and alternative medicine (CAM) [published online ahead of print (February 22, 2018)]. *Psychol Health Med.* February 2018. doi:10.1080/13548506.2018.1442010

133. Park C. Mind-Body CAM Interventions: Current Status and Considerations for Integration Into Clinical Health Psychology. *J Clin Psychol.* 2013;69(1):45-63. doi:10.1002/jclp.21910

134. Owens JE, Menard M. The Quantification of Placebo Effects Within a General Model of Health Care Outcomes. *J Altern Complement Med.* 2011;17(9):817-821. doi:10.1089/acm.2010.0566

135. Lund K, Petersen GL, Erlandsen M, et al. The magnitude of placebo analgesia effects depends on how they are conceptualized. *J Psychosom Res.* 2015;79(6):663-668. doi:10.1016/j.jpsychores.2015.05.002

136. McGrady A, Lynch D, Nagel R, Zsembik C. Application of the high risk model of threat perception to a primary care patient population. *J Nerv Ment Dis.* 1999;187(6):369-375. http://www.ncbi.nlm.nih.gov/pubmed/10379724.

137. Kermit K, Devine DA, Tatman SM. High risk model of threat perception in chronic pain patients: implications for primary care and chronic pain programs. *J Nerv Ment Dis.* 2000;188(9):577-582. http://www.ncbi.nlm.nih.gov/pubmed/11009330.

138. Chaves JF, Brown JM. Spontaneous cognitive strategies for the control of clinical pain and stress. *J Behav Med.* 1987;10(3):263-276. doi:10.1007/BF00846540

139. Polusny MA, Erbes CR, Murdoch M, Arbisi PA, Thuras P, Rath MB. Prospective risk factors for new-onset post-traumatic stress disorder in National Guard soldiers deployed to Iraq. *Psychol Med.* 2011;41(4):687-698. doi:10.1017/S0033291710002047

140. Kehle SM, Ferrier-Auerbach AG, Meis LA, Arbisi PA, Erbes CR, Polusny MA. Predictors of postdeployment alcohol use disorders in National Guard soldiers deployed to Operation Iraqi Freedom. *Psychol Addict Behav.* 2012;26(1):42-50. doi:10.1037/a0024663

141. Ferrier-Auerbach AG, Erbes CR, Polusny MA, Rath CM, Sponheim SR. Predictors of emotional distress reported by soldiers in the combat zone. *J Psychiatr Res.* 2010;44(7):470-476. doi:10.1016/j.jpsychires.2009.10.010

142. Ferrier-Auerbach AG, Kehle SM, Erbes CR, Arbisi PA, Thuras P, Polusny MA. Predictors of alcohol use prior to deployment in National Guard Soldiers. *Addict Behav.* 2009;34(8):625-631. doi:10.1016/j.addbeh.2009.03.027

143. Erbes CR, Kaler ME, Schult T, Polusny MA, Arbisi PA. Mental health diagnosis and occupational functioning in National Guard/Reserve veterans returning from Iraq. *J Rehabil Res Dev.* 2011;48(10):1159. doi:10.1682/JRRD.2010.11.0212

144. Meis LA, Barry RA, Kehle SM, Erbes CR, Polusny MA. Relationship adjustment, PTSD symptoms, and treatment utilization among coupled National Guard soldiers deployed to Iraq. *J Fam Psychol.* 2010;24(5):560-567. doi:10.1037/a0020925

145. Erbes CR, Meis LA, Polusny MA, Compton JS. Couple adjustment and

posttraumatic stress disorder symptoms in National Guard veterans of the Iraq war. *J Fam Psychol.* 2011;25(4):479-487. doi:10.1037/a0024007

146. Gewirtz AH, Polusny MA, DeGarmo DS, Khaylis A, Erbes CR. Posttraumatic stress symptoms among National Guard soldiers deployed to Iraq: Associations with parenting behaviors and couple adjustment. *J Consult Clin Psychol.* 2010;78(5):599-610. doi:10.1037/a0020571

147. Arbisi PA, Polusny MA, Erbes CR, Thuras P, Reddy MK. The Minnesota Multiphasic Personality Inventory–2 Restructured Form in National Guard soldiers screening positive for posttraumatic stress disorder and mild traumatic brain injury. *Psychol Assess.* 2011;23(1):203-214. doi:10.1037/a0021339

148. Arbisi PA, Rusch L, Polusny MA, Thuras P, Erbes CR. Does cynicism play a role in failure to obtain needed care? Mental health service utilization among returning U.S. National Guard soldiers. *Psychol Assess.* 2013;25(3):991-996. doi:10.1037/a0032225

149. Kehle SM, Polusny MA, Murdoch M, et al. Early mental health treatment-seeking among U.S. National Guard soldiers deployed to Iraq. *J Trauma Stress.* 2010;23(1):n/a-n/a. doi:10.1002/jts.20480

150. Murray CJL, Vos T, Lozano R, et al. Disability-adjusted life years (DALYs) for 291 diseases and injuries in 21 regions, 1990-2010: A systematic analysis for the Global Burden of Disease Study 2010. *Lancet.* 2012;380(9859):2197-2223. doi:10.1016/S0140-6736(12)61689-4

151. Nahin RL. Severe Pain in Veterans: The Effect of Age and Sex, and Comparisons With the General Population. *J Pain.* 2017;18(3):247-254. doi:10.1016/j.jpain.2016.10.021

152. Lew HL, Otis JD, Tun C, Kerns RD, Clark ME, Cifu DX. Prevalence of chronic pain, posttraumatic stress disorder, and persistent postconcussive symptoms in OIF/OEF veterans: polytrauma clinical triad. *J Rehabil Res Dev.* 2009;46(6):697-702. doi:10.1682/JRRD.2009.01.0006

153. Outcalt SD, Kroenke K, Krebs EE, et al. Chronic pain and comorbid mental health conditions: independent associations of posttraumatic stress disorder and depression with pain, disability, and quality of life. *J Behav Med.* 2015;38(3):535-543. doi:10.1007/s10865-015-9628-3

154. Seal KH, Bertenthal D, Barnes DE, et al. Association of Traumatic Brain Injury With Chronic Pain in Iraq and Afghanistan Veterans: Effect of Comorbid Mental Health Conditions. *Arch Phys Med Rehabil.* 2017;98(8):1636-1645. doi:10.1016/j.apmr.2017.03.026

155. Toblin RL, Quartana PJ, Riviere LA, Walper KC, Hoge CW. Chronic pain and opioid use in US soldiers after combat deployment. *JAMA Intern Med.* 2014;174(8):1400. doi:10.1001/jamainternmed.2014.2726

156. Clarke TC, Nahin RL. Use of Complementary Health Approaches for

Musculoskeletal Pain Disorders Among Adults: United States, 2012. *Natl Heal Stat Rep*. 2016;(No.98):1-8. https://www.cdc.gov/nchs/data/nhsr/nhsr098.pdf.

157. Cramer H, Ward L, Saper R, Fishbein D, Dobos G, Lauche R. The safety of yoga: A systematic review and meta-analysis of randomized controlled trials. *Am J Epidemiol*. 2015;182(4):281-293. doi:10.1093/aje/kwv071

158. Franklin GM. Opioids for chronic noncancer pain: A position paper of the American Academy of Neurology. *Neurology*. 2014;83(14):1277-1284. doi:10.1212/WNL.0000000000000839

159. Qaseem A, Wilt TJ, McLean RM, Forciea MA. Noninvasive treatments for acute, subacute, and chronic low back pain: A clinical practice guideline from the American College of Physicians. *Ann Intern Med*. 2017;166(7):514-530. doi:10.7326/M16-2367

160. Lee C, Crawford C, Schoomaker E. Movement Therapies for the Self-Management of Chronic Pain Symptoms. *Pain Med*. 2014;15(S1):S40-S53. doi:10.1111/pme.12411

161. Chou R, Deyo R, Friedly J, et al. Nonpharmacologic therapies for low back pain: A systematic review for an American College of physicians clinical practice guideline. *Ann Intern Med*. 2017;166(7):493-505. doi:10.7326/M16-2459

162. Kligler B, Bair MJ, Banerjea R, et al. Clinical Policy Recommendations from the VHA State-of-the-Art Conference on Non-Pharmacological Approaches to Chronic Musculoskeletal Pain. *J Gen Intern Med*. 2018;(November). doi:10.1007/s11606-018-4323-z

163. Bair M, Wu J. Association of Depression and Anxiety Alone and in Combination with Chronic Musculoskeletal Pain in Primary Care Patients. *Psychosom ....* 2008;70(8):890-897. doi:10.1097/PSY.0b013e318185c510.Association

164. Kroenke K, Outcalt S, Krebs E, et al. Association between anxiety, health-related quality of life and functional impairment in primary care patients with chronic pain. *Gen Hosp Psychiatry*. 2013;35(4):359-365. doi:10.1016/j.genhosppsych.2013.03.020

165. Miller S, Gaylord S, Buben A, et al. Literature Review of Research on Chronic Pain and Yoga in Military Populations. *Medicines*. 2017;4(3):64. doi:10.3390/medicines4030064

166. Elwy AR, Groessl EJ, Eisen S V., et al. A Systematic Scoping Review of Yoga Intervention Components and Study Quality. *Am J Prev Med*. 2014;47(2):220-232. doi:10.1016/j.amepre.2014.03.012

167. Goertz C, Marriott BP, Finch MD, et al. Military Report More Complementary and Alternative Medicine Use than Civilians. *J Altern Complement Med*. 2013;19(6):509-517. doi:10.1089/acm.2012.0108

168. Groessl EJ, Liu L, Chang DG, et al. Yoga for Military Veterans with Chronic Low Back Pain: A Randomized Clinical Trial. *Am J Prev Med.* 2017;53(5):599-608. doi:10.1016/j.amepre.2017.05.019
169. Quilty MT, Saper RB, Goldstein R, Khalsa SBS. Yoga in the Real World: Perceptions, Motivators, Barriers, and Patterns of Use. *Glob Adv Heal Med.* 2013;2(1):44-49. doi:10.7453/gahmj.2013.2.1.008
170. Park CL, Riley KE, Bedesin E, Stewart VM. Why practice yoga? Practitioners' motivations for adopting and maintaining yoga practice. *J Health Psychol.* 2016;21(6):887-896. doi:10.1177/1359105314541314
171. Stussman BJ, Black LI, Barnes PM, Clarke TC, Nahin RL. Wellness-related Use of Common Complementary Health Approaches Among Adults: United States, 2012. *Natl Health Stat Report.* 2015;(85):1-12. https://www.cdc.gov/nchs/data/nhsr/nhsr085.pdf.
172. Dillman DA, Smyth JD, Christian LM. *Internet, Phone, Mail, and Mixed-Mode Surveys: The Tailored Design Method.* 4th ed. Hoboken, NJ: Wiley; 2014.
173. Von Korff M. Assessment of Chronic Pain in Epidemiological and Health Services Research: Empirical Bases and New Directions. In: Turk DC, Melzack R, eds. *Handbook of Pain Assessment.* Third edit. New York, New York: Guilford Press; 2011:455-473. https://www.guilford.com/books/Handbook-of-Pain-Assessment/Turk-Melzack/9781606239766.
174. Pilkonis PA, Choi SW, Reise SP, et al. Item banks for measuring emotional distress from the Patient-Reported Outcomes Measurement Information System (PROMIS®): depression, anxiety, and anger. *Assessment.* 2011;18(3):263-283. doi:10.1177/1073191111411667
175. Rosenbaum P, Rubin D. The central role of the propensity score in observational studies for causal effects. *Biometrika.* 1983;70(1):41-55. doi:10.1093/biomet/70.1.41
176. StataCorp. Stata Statistical Software: Release 15. 2017.
177. Rubin DB. Using Propensity Scores to Help Design Observational Studies: Application to the Tobacco Litigation. *Heal Serv Outcomes Res Methodol.* 2001;2(3/4):169-188. doi:10.1023/A:1020363010465
178. Leuven E, Sianesi B. PSMATCH2: Stata module to perform full Mahalnobis and propensity score matching, common support graphing, and covariate imbalance testing (version 4.0.12). 2003. http://ideas/repec.org/c/boc/bocode/s432001.html.
179. IOM (Institute of Medicine), A. Pizzo P, M. Clark N, Carter Pokras O. *Relieving Pain in America: A Blueprint for Transforming Prevention, Care, Education, and Research.* Washington, DC; 2011. doi:10.3109/15360288.2012.678473

180. Schoomaker EB, Buckenmaier CC. For the Relief of Suffering. *J Gen Intern Med*. 2018:7-8. doi:10.1007/s11606-018-4364-3
181. Kerns RD, Krebs EE, Atkins D. Making Integrated Multimodal Pain Care a Reality: A Path Forward. *J Gen Intern Med*. 2018:2-4. doi:10.1007/s11606-018-4361-6
182. Taylor SL, Elwy AR. Complementary and Alternative Medicine for US Veterans and Active Duty Military Personnel. *Med Care*. 2014;52(12 Suppl 5):S1-S4. doi:10.1097/MLR.0000000000000270
183. Becker WC, DeBar LL, Heapy AA, et al. A Research Agenda for Advancing Non-pharmacological Management of Chronic Musculoskeletal Pain: Findings from a VHA State-of-the-art Conference. *J Gen Intern Med*. 2018. doi:10.1007/s11606-018-4345-6
184. Ward L, Stebbings S, Cherkin D, Baxter GD. Yoga for Functional Ability, Pain and Psychosocial Outcomes in Musculoskeletal Conditions: A Systematic Review and Meta-Analysis. *Musculoskeletal Care*. 2013;11(4):203-217. doi:10.1002/msc.1042
185. Büssing A, Ostermann T, Lüdtke R, Michalsen A. Effects of yoga interventions on pain and pain-associated disability: A meta-analysis. *J Pain*. 2012;13(1):1-9. doi:10.1016/j.jpain.2011.10.001
186. Clarke TC, Black LI, Stussman BJ, Barnes PM, Nahin RL. Trends in the use of complementary health approaches among adults: United States, 2002-2012. *Natl Health Stat Report*. 2015;(79):1-16.
187. Ipsos Public Affairs. *2016 Yoga in America Study*.; 2016. http://media.yogajournal.com/wp-content/uploads/2016-Yoga-in-America-Study-Comprehensive-RESULTS.pdf.
188. Tick H, Nielsen A, Pelletier KR, et al. Evidence-Based Nonpharmacologic Strategies for Comprehensive Pain Care. *EXPLORE*. March 2018. doi:10.1016/j.explore.2018.02.001
189. Combs M a., Thorn BE. Barriers and facilitators to yoga use in a population of individuals with self-reported chronic low back pain: A qualitative approach. *Complement Ther Clin Pract*. 2014;20(4):268-275. doi:10.1016/j.ctcp.2014.07.006
190. Groessl EJ, Liu L, Chang DG, et al. Yoga for Military Veterans with Chronic Low Back Pain: A Randomized Clinical Trial. *Am J Prev Med*. 2017;53(5):599-608. doi:10.1016/j.amepre.2017.05.019
191. Sovik R, Bhavanani AB. History, Philosophy, and Practice of Yoga. In: Khalsa SBS, Cohen L, McCall T, Telles S, eds. *The Principles and Practice of Yoga in Health Care*. Edinburgh, UK: Handspring Publishing; 2016:17-30.
192. Creswell JW, Plano Clark VL. *Designing and Conducting Mixed Methods Research*. Thousand Oaks, CA: Sage Publications; 2011.

193. Krebs EE, Lorenz KA, Bair MJ, et al. Development and Initial Validation of the PEG, a Three-item Scale Assessing Pain Intensity and Interference. *J Gen Intern Med.* 2009;24(6):733-738. doi:10.1007/s11606-009-0981-1

194. Von Korff M, Scher AI, Helmick C, et al. United States National Pain Strategy for Population Research: Concepts, Definitions, and Pilot Data. *J Pain.* 2016;17(10):1068-1080. doi:10.1016/j.jpain.2016.06.009

195. Selim AJ, Rogers W, Fleishman JA, et al. Updated U.S. population standard for the Veterans RAND 12-item Health Survey (VR-12). *Qual Life Res.* 2009;18(1):43-52. doi:10.1007/s11136-008-9418-2

196. Jones D, Kazis L, Lee A, et al. Health status assessments using the Veterans SF-12 and SF-36: methods for evaluating otucomes in the Veterans Health Administration. *J Ambul Care Manag.* 2001;24(3):68-86. doi:10.1097/00004479-200107000-00011

197. QSR International Pty Ltd. NVivo qualitative data analysis software. 2012.

198. Saldaña J. *The Coding Manual for Qualitative Researchers.* Second edi. Thousand Oaks, CA: SAGE; 2013.

199. Davies D, Dodd J. Qualitative Research and the Question of Rigor. *Qual Health Res.* 2002;12(2):279-289. doi:10.1177/104973230201200211

200. Miles MB, Huberman AM, Saldaña J. *Qualitative Data Analysis.* 3rd ed. Thousand Oaks, CA: SAGE Publications; 2014.

201. Schulz-Heik RJ, Meyer H, Mahoney L, et al. Results from a clinical yoga program for veterans: Yoga via telehealth provides comparable satisfaction and health improvements to in-person yoga. *BMC Complement Altern Med.* 2017;17(1):1-9. doi:10.1186/s12906-017-1705-4

202. Saper RB. Minding the Mat: Moving the Yoga Field Forward. *Glob Adv Heal Med.* 2015;4(3):5-6. doi:10.7453/gahmj.2015.054

203. National Center for Complementary and Integrative Health. *Complementary, Alternative, or Integrative Health: What's In a Name?*; 2016. https://nccih.nih.gov/health/integrative-health. Accessed January 2, 2018.

204. National Center for Complementary and Integrative Health. Use of Complementary Health Approaches in the U.S.: National Health Interview Survey (NHIS). https://nccih.nih.gov/research/statistics/NHIS/2012/key-findings. Published 2017. Accessed February 1, 2018.

205. Quandt SA, Verhoef MJ, Arcury TA, et al. Development of an international questionnaire to measure use of complementary and alternative medicine (I-CAM-Q). *J Altern Complement Med.* 2009;15(4):331-339. doi:10.1089/acm.2008.0521

206. National Center for Complementary and Integrative Health. 2016 Strategic Plan: Exploring the Science of Complementary and Integrative Health. NIH

Publication No. 16-AT-7643. https://nccih.nih.gov/sites/nccam.nih.gov/files/NCCIH_2016_Strategic_Plan.pdf. Published 2016. Accessed February 7, 2018.

207. Stussman BJ, Bethell CD, Gray C, Nahin RL. Development of the adult and child complementary medicine questionnaires fielded on the National Health Interview Survey. *BMC Complement Altern Med.* 2013;13(1):328. doi:10.1186/1472-6882-13-328

208. Eisenberg DM, Kessler RC, Foster C, Norlock FE, Calkins DR, Delbanco TL. Unconventional Medicine in the United States -- Prevalence, Costs, and Patterns of Use. *N Engl J Med.* 1993;328(4):246-252. doi:10.1056/NEJM199301283280406

209. Bishop FL, Lewith GT. Who uses CAM a narrative review of demographic characteristics and health factors associated with CAM use. *Evidence-based Complement Altern Med.* 2010;7(1):11-28. doi:10.1093/ecam/nen023

210. Healthcare Analysis & Information Group. Veterans Health Administration Office of ASDUH for Health Policy and Planning. Department of Veterans Affairs. *FY 2015 VHA Complementary & Integrative Health (CIH) Services.*; 2015.

211. 2012 NHIS Questionnaire - Adult CAM: Adult Alternative Health/Complementary And Alternative Medicine. ftp://ftp.cdc.gov/pub/Health_Statistics/NCHS/Survey_Questionnaires/NHIS/2012/English/qalthealt.pdf. Accessed March 26, 2018.

212. Willis GB. Cognitive Interviewing: A "how to" guide. In: *1999 Meeting of the American Statistical Association.* http://www.chime.ucla.edu/publications/docs/cognitive interviewing guide.pdf.

213. Willis G. *Cognitive Interviewing.* Thousand Oaks, CA: SAGE Publications, Inc.; 2005. doi:10.4135/9781412983655

214. Patient-Reported Outcomes Measurement Information System. *PROMIS Scoring Guide: Version 1.0 Short Forms.*; 2011. https://www.assessmentcenter.net/documents/PROMIS Scoring Manual-CATs, Profiles, Short Forms.pdf.

215. Muller CJ, Maclehose RF. Estimating predicted probabilities from logistic regression: Different methods correspond to different target populations. *Int J Epidemiol.* 2014;43(3):962-970. doi:10.1093/ije/dyu029

216. Raghunathan TE, Lepkowski JM, Van Hoewyk J, Solenberger P. A multivariate technique for multiply imputing missing values using a sequence of regression models. *Surv Methodol.* 2001;27(1):85-95.

217. Van Buuren S, Brand JPL, Groothuis-Oudshoorn CGM, Rubin DB. Fully conditional specification in multivariate imputation. *J Stat Comput Simul.*

2006;76(12):1049-1064. doi:10.1080/10629360600810434

218. Rubin DB. Inference and missing data. *Biometrika*. 1976;63(3):581-592. doi:10.1093/biomet/63.3.581

219. Morris TP, White IR, Royston P. Tuning multiple imputation by predictive mean matching and local residual draws. *BMC Med Res Methodol*. 2014;14(1). doi:10.1186/1471-2288-14-75

220. Little RJA. Missing-Data Adjustments in Large Surveys. *J Bus Econ Stat*. 1988;6(3):287-296. doi:10.2307/1391881

221. Peregoy JA, Clarke TC, Jones LI, Stussman BJ, Nahin RL. Regional Variation in Use of Complementary Health Approaches by U.S. Adults. *NCHS Data Brief*. 2015;April(146):1-8. doi:10.1038/nbt.3121.ChIP-nexus

222. Herman PM, Sorbero ME, Sims-Columbia AC. Complementary and Alternative Medicine Services in the Military Health System. 2017;23(11):837-843. doi:10.1089/acm.2017.0236

223. Crawford C, Lee C, Freilich D. Effectiveness of Active Self-Care Complementary and Integrative Medicine Therapies: Options for the Management of Chronic Pain Symptoms. *Pain Med*. 2014;15(S1):S86-S95. doi:10.1111/pme.12407

224. Park CL, Finkelstein-Fox L, Barnes DM, Mazure CM, Hoff R. CAM use in recently-returned OEF/OIF/OND US veterans: Demographic and psychosocial predictors. *Complement Ther Med*. 2016;28:50-56. doi:10.1016/j.ctim.2016.08.004

225. Department of Veterans Affairs. National Center for Veterans Analysis and Statistics. VA Utilization Profile FY2016. https://www.va.gov/vetdata/docs/Quickfacts/VA_Utilization_Profile.pdf. Published 2017. Accessed February 5, 2018.

226. Davis MT, Mulvaney-Day N, Larson MJ, Hoover R, Mauch D. Complementary and Alternative Medicine Among Veterans and Military Personnel. *Med Care*. 2014;52(12 Suppl 5):S83-S90. doi:10.1097/MLR.0000000000000227

227. Elwy RA, Johnston JM, Bormann JE, Hull A, Taylor SL. A systematic scoping review of complementary and alternative medicine mind and body practices to improve the health of veterans and military personnel. *Med Care*. 2014;52(12):S70-S82. doi:10.1097/MLR.0000000000000228